Intelligent Perception and Information Processing

This book series Intelligent Perception and Information Processing is grounded in artificial intelligence and signal and information processing theory, focusing on key technologies such as communication, vision, and location for signal and information perception, processing, transmission, and storage. It is committed to solving key and difficult problems in wireless perception, machine vision, information and coding, image processing, multi-source information fusion, environment configurable intelligent transmission, cross-media transmission, knowledge graph and other application areas, and promoting the development of intelligent perception and signal processing.

Yao Ding · Zhili Zhang · Haojie Hu ·
Renxiang Guan · Jie Feng · Zhiyong Lv

Graph Neural Network for Hyperspectral Image Clustering

Science Press
Beijing

Springer

Yao Ding
Xi'an Research Institute of High Technology
Xi'an, Shaanxi, China

Haojie Hu
Xi'an Research Institute of High Technology
Xi'an, Shaanxi, China

Jie Feng
School of Artificial Intelligence
Xidian University
Xi'an, Shaanxi, China

Zhili Zhang
Xi'an Research Institute of High Technology
Xi'an, Shaanxi, China

Renxiang Guan
National University of Defense Technology
Changsha, Hunan, China

Zhiyong Lv
School of computer science and engineering
Xi'an University of Technology
Xi'an, Shaanxi, China

ISSN 3059-3808 ISSN 3059-3816 (electronic)
Intelligent Perception and Information Processing
ISBN 978-981-96-7709-2 ISBN 978-981-96-7710-8 (eBook)
https://doi.org/10.1007/978-981-96-7710-8

Jointly published with Science Press
The print edition is not for sale in China mainland. Customers from China mainland please order the print book from: Science Press.

This Springer imprint is published by the registered company Springer Nature Singapore Pte Ltd.
The registered company address is: 152 Beach Road, #21-01/04 Gateway East, Singapore 189721, Singapore

Preface

Hyperspectral image (HSI) classification holds significant strategic value in the military domain. By capturing continuous spectral information across hundreds of narrow bands from ground objects, it enables high-precision identification and dynamic monitoring of battlefield environments, military installations, and camouflaged targets. In military remote sensing applications, this technology can penetrate traditional camouflage methods to accurately detect concealed equipment, underground facilities, or spectrally disguised military assets, providing multidimensional intelligence support for battlefield reconnaissance. For instance, leveraging unique spectral "fingerprints" of materials allows differentiation between decoys and real targets or detection of chemical weapon residues. This classification capability not only enhances the timeliness and accuracy of battlefield situational awareness but also strengthens the stealth and strike efficiency of military operations. It serves as a crucial technological foundation for establishing comprehensive battlefield transparency systems and implementing precision warfare, emerging as a core component in securing information dominance within modern informatized warfare paradigms.

Hyperspectral imaging has emerged as a transformative technology in remote sensing, capturing intricate spectral-spatial information across hundreds of narrow and contiguous bands. This wealth of data enables unprecedented precision in applications ranging from environmental monitoring and agricultural management to mineral exploration and military reconnaissance. However, the high dimensionality, spectral variability, and complex spatial structures inherent to hyperspectral images present formidable challenges for traditional clustering methods. The scarcity of labeled data further underscores the need for robust unsupervised learning techniques capable of extracting meaningful patterns from unannotated HSI datasets. This monograph, *Graph Neural Network for Hyperspectral Image Clustering*, addresses these challenges by exploring cutting-edge graph-based learning frameworks tailored for HSI analysis. Traditional clustering algorithms, such as k-means and subspace clustering, often falter due to their reliance on linear assumptions or inability to model the non-Euclidean relationships between pixels. In contrast, graph learning provides a natural paradigm to encode spatial-spectral dependencies, leveraging the topological structure of HSI data to enhance clustering accuracy and robustness.

The motivation for this work stems from two converging trends: the exponential growth of hyperspectral data from advanced sensors and satellites, and the rapid maturation of graph-based deep learning frameworks. This intersection presents a timely opportunity to redefine clustering methodologies, moving beyond Euclidean assumptions to embrace the graph-structured nature of HSI. Furthermore, this endeavor is inherently interdisciplinary, weaving together insights from machine learning, computer vision, and geospatial sciences to address real-world challenges. The book begins with a comprehensive review of classical and deep learning-based clustering methods, critically analyzing their limitations in handling HSI's spectral complexity and spatial heterogeneity. It then introduces a series of innovative graph-based frameworks that integrate advanced techniques such as graph neural networks (GNNs), contrastive learning, and multi-view fusion. The main research content of this book is summarized as follows: Chapter 1 mainly introduces the research background of this book, explains the practical significance, and outlines the current situation and existing problems of hyperspectral remote sensing image clustering. Furthermore, the research content and chapter arrangement of this book are specifically presented. Chapter 2 proposes a novel framework that mines hard samples and enforces consistency between spatial and spectral views to improve discriminative feature learning. Chapter 3 focuses on harmonizing texture and spectral-spatial features through contrastive learning and adaptive affinity matrix fusion. Chapter 4 introduces a computationally efficient approach that denoises graph structures using low-pass filters and enhances robustness through cross-view contrastive learning. Chapter 5 addresses the poor robustness, adaptability, and feature presentation of existing methods adopting self-supervised graph convolutional with locality preserving low-pass embedding. Chapter 6 proposed an adaptive homophily structure graph clustering method using structural information of HSI. Each chapter systematically builds on prior concepts, offering theoretical insights, algorithmic details, and experimental validation on benchmark datasets such as Salinas, Pavia University, and Trento. The results demonstrate significant improvements in clustering accuracy, scalability, and noise resilience compared to state-of-the-art methods.

This monograph is designed for researchers, practitioners, and graduate students in remote sensing, machine learning, and data science. While a foundational understanding of machine learning and image processing is assumed, the text provides clear explanations of graph theory, contrastive learning, and subspace clustering to ensure accessibility. By bridging the gap between graph-structured data analysis and hyperspectral imaging, this work not only advances the field of unsupervised learning but also offers practical tools for real-world applications.

We hope this monograph inspires further innovation in graph-based learning for remote sensing, fostering solutions that unlock the full potential of hyperspectral data in addressing global environmental and societal challenges.

Xi'an, China — Yao Ding
Xi'an, China — Zhili Zhang
Xi'an, China — Haojie Hu
Changsha, China — Renxiang Guan
Xi'an, China — Jie Feng
Xi'an, China — Zhiyong Lv

Contents

Chapter 1
Introduction

1.1 Background and Significance of Hyperspectral Image Clustering

Hyperspectral image (HSI) has gained significant attention in the field of remote sensing and image analysis. Unlike traditional multispectral imaging, which captures images in a few broad spectral bands, hyperspectral imaging captures data across a wide range of the electromagnetic spectrum, often hundreds of contiguous spectral bands. This rich spectral information allows for more detailed and precise analysis of the materials and objects within an image [1]. HSI finds wide application in various fields, such as mineral exploration [2], bioinformatics [3], and aerial reconnaissance [4]. However, the interpretation of HSI data frequently requires a substantial number of high-quality labeled samples to prevent under-fitting due to insufficient training data. In practice, the process of collecting and labeling these samples is laborious, expensive, time-consuming, and often inefficient. Moreover, in certain hazardous or complex environments, obtaining training samples can be particularly challenging, which significantly limits the practical applications of HSI. Consequently, there is a pressing need to develop unsupervised learning mechanisms to enhance the analysis and utilization of hyperspectral image.

Clustering is a powerful unsupervised technique for pattern recognition and information extraction, and it is widely used for the interpretation of hyperspectral imaging (HSI) data [5]. This method groups similar pixels and segregates dissimilar ones, with each cluster representing a distinct class. By thoroughly exploiting the structural properties of hyperspectral data based on a similarity criterion, clustering enables the identification and categorization of different materials and objects within the image [6]. However, hyperspectral image has a significantly more intricate internal structure compared to handwritten figures, text, natural images, and multispectral images. Additionally, HSIs exhibit substantial spectral variability, as pixels belonging to the same class can have different spectral signatures due to the complexity of the

Y. Ding et al., *Graph Neural Network for Hyperspectral Image Clustering*, Intelligent Perception and Information Processing, https://doi.org/10.1007/978-981-96-7710-8_1

imaging environment. Consequently, hyperspectral image clustering presents a more challenging task.

Hyperspectral image clustering typically encompasses two primary tasks: estimating the number of clusters and constructing an appropriate clustering model. However, the first task is not the core of hyperspectral image clustering, and is relatively limited within the hyperspectral clustering community. In practice, the number of clusters is often set based on the known number of classes in the ground truth data [7]. As for the second task, the reasonability and effectiveness of clustering model directly influence the final clustering accuracy. Therefore, the development and refinement of clustering methodologies and models have been a central focus in the field of hyperspectral image (HSI) processing. Most existing work in this area has concentrated on improving clustering techniques, exploring various algorithms, and integrating advanced methods to enhance performance. In this book, we also place significant emphasis on clustering models and methods.

1.2 Research Status and Existing Problems

1.2.1 Traditional Hyperspectral Image Clustering Methods and Existing Problems

Traditional clustering methods for hyperspectral image have been widely studied and applied due to their effectiveness in unsupervised pattern recognition and information extraction. Traditional clustering methods, such as K-means [8], commonly rely on pairwise distance metrics, like the Euclidean distance, to measure similarity. However, due to issues such as mixed pixels and redundant spectral bands [9], these methods often produce unreliable measurements, significantly complicating the task of hyperspectral image (HSI) clustering. Subspace clustering [10] is another classical approach for hyperspectral image clustering, as its ability to handle high-dimensional data and its reliable performance. Technically, subspace clustering aims to represent data points as linear combinations of a self-expressive dictionary within the same subspace [11]. The process typically involves two main steps: self-representation [12] and spectral clustering (SC) [13]. To enhance the performance of subspace clustering, numerous studies have focused on constructing a robust affinity matrix using various techniques. However, traditional subspace clustering models are often based on Euclidean data, which can lead to the neglect of the inherent graph-structured information present in hyperspectral image data points.

However, the spatial information encapsulated within HSI is also crucial. This implies that relying solely on the spectral information of HSI is insufficient. Consequently, to fully leverage the spectral-spatial information of HSI and enhance clustering accuracy, various spectral-spatial HSI clustering methods have been developed, which have demonstrated superior performance compared to those that rely exclusively on spectral information. A typical example is the spectral-spatial sparse subspace clustering (SSC) algorithm [14]. It promotes the target pixels to be represented by highly related atoms via a weighting strategy and incorporates the spatial neighborhood information to generate an integrated self-representation model by constructing an eight-neighborhood local average spatial regularization. In addition, in [15], a spectral-spatial SSC based on 3D edge-preserving filtering (SSC-3DEPF) algorithm was put forward. It utilizes 3D edge-preserving filtering for the sparse coefficient matrix obtained by SSC to extract the spectral-spatial information to generate a more accurate coefficient matrix, which is favorable for clustering. Unfortunately, the aforementioned methods are shallow classifiers based on the handcrafted feature or raw feature spaces, which cannot learn the high-level features of HSI and are not suitable for characterizing the large spectral variability and the complex internal structure of HSI datasets effectively [16].

1.2.2 Hyperspectral Image Clustering Methods Based on Deep Learning and Existing Problems

Recent advancements in machine learning, particularly deep learning, have also influenced hyperspectral image clustering. Convolutional Neural Networks (CNNs) have been adapted to perform dimensionality reduction and clustering tasks directly on hyperspectral data. These methods have demonstrated impressive performance in automatically learning relevant features from raw hyperspectral images, often outperforming traditional approaches. Since there are no available labeled samples, these models are generally optimized in an unsupervised way. According to different unsupervised learning mechanism, deep learning-based clustering methods can be further divided into three main categories: autoencoder-based clustering; generative network-based clustering; contractive learning-based clustering.

Autoencoder-based clustering include an encoder for data representation and a decoder for reconstruction, training by minimizing reconstruction errors. A prominent example is the deep clustering network (DCN) [17], which employs a deep autoencoder for dimensionality reduction to extract features more compatible with k-means clustering, integrating both dimensionality reduction and clustering within a single framework. Furthermore, a spatial–spectral subspace clustering network (DS3C-Net) was designed by Lei et al. [18] to extract spatial–spectral features by collaborative constraint and the multiscale autoencoder. Unlike autoencoder-based clustering, generative network-based methods focus on accurately capturing the true data structure to produce high-quality samples, enhancing feature discriminability. The most notable approaches are based on Generative Adversarial Networks (GANs), which consist of a generator and a discriminator. These components improve feature quality through adversarial interactions. A typical example is categorical GAN (CatGAN) [19], which employs a min–max adversarial game to learn an unsupervised discriminative classifier by balancing mutual information between observations and predicted class distributions. Based on the CatGAN, in [20], an information-maximizing GAN (InfoGAN) was proposed. It enhances the clustering performance by exploiting the mutual information among the fixed small subset of latent variables and the observations. In addition to GAN-based models, a set of contrastive learning-based clustering methods has been developed, leveraging on pulling similar instances closer together in the feature space while pushing dissimilar ones apart, thereby improving the discriminative power of the learned representations. For example, Cai et al. [21] presented a neighborhood contrastive subspace clustering (NCSC) network, a scalable and robust DSC approach, for unsupervised classification of large hyperspectral images. Furthermore, Hou et al. [22] introduced contrast learning into HSI features learning, and the unlabeled samples were utilized to alleviate the label information insufficient problem.

Deep learning-based clustering methods achieve higher accuracy by leveraging their robust feature extraction and nonlinear modeling abilities, making them a prominent focus in clustering research. Nevertheless, the aforementioned methods are not designed specifically for large-scale HSI clustering, and the clustering performance on complex large-scale HSI dataset clustering should be improved. In addition, due to labeled data deficiency, large spectral variability, and high dimension of HSIs, most of the existing deep clustering methods cannot effectively learn remarkable and adaptive high-level features for HSI clustering, which leads to poor clustering accuracy. Finally, most of the deep clustering methods ignore the layer-wise local features, which results in poor adaptability to different HSI datasets.

1.2.3 Graph-Based Hyperspectral Image Clustering Methods

Graph-based clustering is a recently developed advanced approach for hyperspectral image clustering, rooted in graph theory. These methods typically represent the relationships among hyperspectral pixels using an adjacency matrix, also known as a similarity graph. Each element of this matrix quantifies the similarity between a pair of pixels or the penalty for separating them into different subgraphs. The adjacency matrix forms the foundation of graph clustering, and its quality significantly influences the final clustering accuracy. Graph-based clustering methods can essentially be regarded as graph cut techniques, which segment a graph into several disjoint and distinctive subgraphs by maximizing the intrasubgraph similarity and minimizing the intersubgraph similarity, with each subgraph denoting a specific class. A typical example is spectral clustering (SC) [23] which generally employs the normalized cut algorithm to conduct graph cutting. Based on spectral clustering, a novel Schrodinger Eigen map with nondiagonal potentials for a spectral–spatial clustering (SENP) algorithm was proposed for HSIs in [24]. In addition, in [25], a graph-based nonlocal total variation (NLTV) method was developed and obtains accurate clustering results for HSIs. Furthermore, a joint spectral–spatial clustering with a block-diagonal amplified affinity matrix (JC-BAAM) algorithm was proposed for better performance by increasing the separability between different classes [26].

In summary, graph-based clustering methods have gained significant attention in hyperspectral clustering due to their flexible graph construction, strong structure information mining capabilities, and relatively robust performance. However, they face challenges such as high computational complexity, requiring a balance between accuracy and efficiency. Additionally, limitations in accurately capturing pixel interactions during graph construction, coupled with spectral variability and high pixel correlations, hinder their ability to fully exploit underlying adjacency relationships, thereby constraining clustering performance. Inspired by the rapid development and wide application of deep learning, it is necessary to develop the graph-based clustering methods based on deep learning techniques to learn the high-level features of HSI and characterizing the large spectral variability and the complex internal structure of HSI datasets effectively. Therefore, we aim to explore the potential application of graph learning for hyperspectral image clustering in this book.

1.3 Research Content and Chapter Arrangement

In this book, the graph learning methods are designed to solve the problems and challenges faced by hyperspectral image clustering and improve classification accuracy, focusing on model construction, improving graph information dissemination methods, and improving composition quality. Multiple graph learning-based hyperspectral image clustering methods are proposed. The research content can be summarized into the following aspects:

Chapter 1. Introduction

This chapter mainly introduces the research background of this book, explains the practical significance of hyperspectral image classification, and reviews the research status and existing problems of hyperspectral image classification. To facilitate the understanding of this book, the basic knowledge of graph networks and the evaluation indicators used in the experiment were introduced. Finally, the research content and chapter arrangement of this book were specifically presented.

Chapter 2. Spatial-Spectral Graph Contrastive with Hard Sample Mining for Hyperspectral Image Clustering

Hyperspectral image (HSI) clustering is a fundamental yet challenging task that groups image pixels with similar features into distinct clusters. Among various approaches, contrastive learning methods, which employ the concept of encouraging semantically similar samples to move closer together while pushing semantically inconsistent samples apart, have garnered significant attention due to their promising performance. However, the most prevalent approaches face two major limitations: 1) treating all samples indiscriminately during optimization, where the abundance of well-categorized samples overwhelms the feature learning process and 2) tending to introduce noise when constructing positive sample pairs through view augmentation or searching the nearest neighbors, which would cause semantic drift of sample features. To solve these issues, we propose a graph autoencoder-based deep clustering framework named spatial–spectral graph contrastive clustering with hard sample mining (SSGCC) that constructs spatial–spectral dual views without data augmentation and focuses more on hard samples rather than treating all samples equally with the aid of spatial–spectral features. Concretely, we extract the spectral features and the neighborhood spatial features of the samples as dual branches to avoid the noise caused by data augmentation and develop the cluster-oriented consistency learning to facilitate the exchange of knowledge between the two spectral–spatial perspectives. In addition, we propose a hard sample mining-based contrastive learning scheme with the aid of spatial–spectral features. To better measure the importance of the samples, we combine spatial features and spectral features to calculate the similarity between sample pairs. The weights of hard sample pairs are dynamically up-weight while the easy ones are down-weighting to improve the discriminative capability.

Chapter 3. Multi-view Subspace Graph Convolutional Clustering for Hyperspectral Images

High-dimensional and complex spectral structures make clustering of hyperspectral images (HSI) a challenging task. Subspace clustering has been shown to be an effective approach for addressing this problem. However, current subspace clustering algorithms are mainly designed for a single view and do not fully exploit spatial or texture feature information in HSI. This study proposed a multiview subspace clustering of HSI based on graph convolutional networks. (1) This chapter uses the powerful classification ability of graph convolutional network and the learning ability of topological relationships between nodes to analyze and express the spatial relationship of HSI. (2) Pixel texture and pixel neighbor spatial-spectral information were sent to construct two graph convolutional subspaces. (3) An attention-based fusion module was used to adaptively construct a more discriminative feature map.

Chapter 4. An Efficient Low-pass Contrastive Graph Clustering Network for Hyperspectral Images

Self-supervised hyperspectral image (HSI) clustering remains a fundamental yet challenging task due to the absence of labeled data and the inherent complexity of spatial-spectral interactions. While recent advancements have explored innovative approaches, existing methods face critical limitations in clustering accuracy, feature discriminability, computational efficiency, and robustness to noise, hindering their practical deployment. In this chapter, a self-supervised efficient low-pass contrastive graph clustering (SLCGC) is introduced for HSIs. Our approach begins with homogeneous region generation, which aggregates pixels into spectrally consistent regions to preserve local spatial-spectral coherence while drastically reducing graph complexity. We then construct a structural graph using an adjacency matrix A and introduce a low-pass graph denoising mechanism to suppress high-frequency noise in the graph topology, ensuring stable feature propagation. A dual-branch graph contrastive learning module is developed, where Gaussian noise perturbations generate augmented views through two multilayer perceptrons (MLPs), and a cross-view contrastive loss enforces structural consistency between views to learn noise-invariant representations. Finally, latent embeddings optimized by this process are clustered via K-means.

Chapter 5. Self-supervised Graph Convolutional with Locality Preserving Low-Pass Embedding for Large-Scale Hyperspectral Image Clustering

Due to prior knowledge deficiency, large spectral variability, and high dimension of hyperspectral image (HSI), HSI clustering is extremely a fundamental but challenging task. Deep clustering methods have achieved remarkable success and have attracted increasing attention in unsupervised HSI classification (HSIC). However, the poor robustness, adaptability, and feature presentation limit their practical application to complex large-scale HSI datasets. Thus, this chapter introduces a novel self-supervised locality preserving low-pass graph convolutional embedding method (L2GCC) for large-scale hyperspectral image clustering. Specifically, a spectral-spatial transformation HSI pre-processing mechanism is introduced to learn superpixel-level spectral-spatial features from HSI and reduce the number of graph nodes for subsequent network processing. In addition, locality preserving low-pass graph convolutional embedding autoencoder is proposed, in which the low-pass graph convolution and layer-wise graph attention are designed to extract the smoother features and preserve layer-wise locality features, respectively. Finally, we develop a self-training strategy, in which a self-training clustering objective employs soft labels to supervise the clustering process and obtain appropriate hidden representations for node clustering.

Chapter 6. Adaptive Homophily Clustering for Hyperspectral Image

Hyperspectral image (HSI) clustering is a fundamental yet challenging task that typically operates without training labels. Recent advancements in deep graph clustering methods have shown promise for HSI due to their ability to effectively encode spatial structural information. However, limitations such as inadequate utilization of structural information, poor feature representation, and weak graph update capabilities hinder their performance. In this chapter, we propose an Adaptive Homophily Structure Graph Clustering method (AHSGC) for HSI. Our approach begins with the generation of homogeneous regions to process HSI and construct the initial graph. Next, we design an adaptive filter graph encoder that captures both high and low-frequency features for subsequent processing. We then develop a graph embedding clustering self-training decoder using KL Divergence to generate pseudo-labels for network training. To enhance graph learning, we introduce homophily-enhanced structure learning, which updates the graph based on the clustering task. This involves estimating node connections through orient correlation estimation and dynamically adjusting graph edges via graph edge sparsification. Finally, we implement joint network optimization to facilitate self-training and graph updates, with K-means used to express latent features.

References

1. Li X, Zhang L, You J (2019) Domain transfer learning for hyperspectral image super-resolution. Rem Sens 11:694
2. Kruse FA, Boardman JW, Huntington JF (2003) Comparison of airborne hyperspectral data and EO-1 Hyperion for mineral mapping. IEEE Trans Geosci Rem Sens 41:1388–1400
3. Kong B, Yu H, Du R, Wang Q (2019) Quantitative estimation of biomass of alpine grasslands using hyperspectral remote sensing. Rangel Ecol Manage 72:336–346
4. Shimoni M, Haelterman R, Perneel C (2019) Hypersectral imaging for military and security applications: combining myriad processing and sensing techniques. IEEE Geosci Rem Sens Mag 7:101–117
5. Zhai H, Zhang H, Zhang L, Li P (2019) Total variation regularized collaborative representation clustering with a locally adaptive dictionary for hyperspectral imagery. IEEE Trans Geosci Remote Sens 57(1):166–180
6. Kashima H, Hu J, Ray B, Singh M (2008) K-means clustering of proportional data using L1 distance. In: Proceedings of IEEE international conference on pattern recognition, pp 1–4
7. Zhang L, Zhang L, Du B, You J, Tao D (June2019) Hyperspectral image unsupervised classification by robust manifold matrix factorization. Inf Sci 485:154–169
8. Zhu J, Jiang Z, Evangelidis GD, Zhang C, Pang S, Li Z (2019) Efficient registration of multi-view point sets by K-means clustering. Inf Sci 488:205–218
9. Hu P, Liu X, Cai Y, Cai Z (Mar.2019) Band selection of hyperspectral images using multiobjective optimization-based sparse self-representation. IEEE Geosci Rem Sens Lett 16(3):452–456
10. Vidal R (2011) Subspace clustering. IEEE Signal Process Mag 28(2):52–68
11. Li Q, Liu W, Li L (2018) Affinity learning via a diffusion process for subspace clustering. Pattern Recognit 84:39–50
12. Ji P, Zhang T, Li H, Salzmann M, Reid I (2017) Deep subspace clustering networks. In: Guyon I, Luxburg UV, Bengio S, Wallach H, Fergus R, Vishwanathan S, Garnett R (eds) Proceedings of advances in neural information processing systems. Curran Associates, Red Hook, pp 24–33
13. Wang R, Nie F, Yu W (Nov.2017) Fast spectral clustering with anchor graph for large hyperspectral images. IEEE Geosci Remote Sens Lett 14(11):2003–2007
14. Zhang H, Zhai H, Zhang L, Li P (2016) Spectral-spatial sparse subspace clustering for hyperspectral images. IEEE Trans Geosci Remote Sens 54(6):3672–3684. https://doi.org/10.1109/TGRS.2016.2524557
15. Li A, Qin A, Shang Z, Tang YY (2019) Spectral-spatial sparse subspace clustering based on three-dimensional edge-preserving filtering for hyperspectral image. Int J Pattern Recognit Artif Intell 33(3):1,955,003
16. Nie F, Wang X, Jordan M, Huang H (2016) The constrained Laplacian rank algorithm for graph-based clustering. Proc AAAI Conf Artif Intell 30(1):1–8
17. Yang B, Fu X, Sidiropoulos ND, Hong M (2017) Towards k-means-friendly spaces: simultaneous deep learning and clustering. In: Proceedings of international conference on machine learning (ICML), pp 3861–3870
18. Lei J, Li X, Peng B, Fang L, Ling N, Huang Q (2021) Deep spatialspectral subspace clustering for hyperspectral image. IEEE Trans Circuits Syst Video Technol 31(7):2686–2697
19. Springenberg JT (2015) Unsupervised and semi-supervised learning with categorical generative adversarial networks. arXiv preprint arXiv:1511.06390
20. Chen X, Duan Y, Houthooft R, Schulman J, Sutskever I, Abbeel P (2016) Infogan: Interpretable representation learning by information maximizing generative adversarial nets. In: Proceedings of Advances in Neural Information Processing Systems (NIPS), pp 2172–2180
21. Cai Y et al (2022) Superpixel contracted neighborhood contrastive subspace clustering network for hyperspectral images. IEEE Trans Geosci Remote Sens 60:1–13
22. Hou S, Shi H, Cao X, Zhang X, Jiao L (2022) Hyperspectral imagery classification based on contrastive learning. IEEE Trans Geosci Remote Sens 60:1–13

23. Shi J, Malik J (Aug.2000) Normalized cuts and image segmentation. IEEE Trans Pattern Anal Mach Intell 22(8):888905
24. Cahill ND, Czaja W, Messinger DW (2014) Schroedinger eigenmaps with nondiagonal potentials for spatial-spectral clustering of hyperspectral imagery. In: Proceedings of Alg. Tech. Multispe. Hyperspe. Ultraspe. Image. XX. International Society for Optics and Photonics (ISOP), vol 9088, p 908,804
25. Zhu W et al (2017) Unsupervised classification in hyperspectral imagery with nonlocal total variation and primal-dual hybrid gradient algorithm. IEEE Trans Geosci Remote Sens 55(5):2786–2798
26. Fan L, Messinger DW (2018) Joint spatial–spectral hyperspectral image clustering using block-diagonal amplified affinity matrix. Opt Eng 57(3):033107

Chapter 2
Spatial-Spectral Graph Contrastive with Hard Sample Mining for Hyperspectral Image Clustering

2.1 Introduction

Hyperspectral imaging (HSI) acquires finely resolved spectral signatures of terrestrial objects, offering strong discriminative power while also preserving extensive spatial details about their distribution [1–4]. As a result, this technology has broad utility in fields such as mineral detection [5, 6], agricultural monitoring [7–9], and urban development planning [10, 11]. Nevertheless, interpreting HSI data is challenging due to its high dimensionality, often requiring large volumes of accurately annotated samples to prevent underfitting caused by insufficient classifier training [12]. Manual annotation, however, is labor-intensive and time-consuming, significantly hindering the practical use of HSI. Thus, advancing unsupervised clustering methods is critically important.

Hyperspectral image clustering seeks to extract distinguishing features that enable pixel grouping into meaningful clusters without requiring labeled data [13–18]. Conventional clustering approaches primarily focus on optimizing an objective function to achieve an ideal solution [19–22]. Yet, these techniques often rely on linear assumptions and fail to capture intricate feature representations, limiting their effectiveness in complex HSI scenarios [23]. In recent years, deep graph clustering methods have risen in prominence, leveraging the robust representational capacity of graph neural networks (GNNs) [24–28]. Within self-supervised graph clustering techniques [30–32], contrastive learning has emerged as a particularly effective strategy. This approach creates supervisory signals by pulling positive sample pairs closer in feature space while pushing negative pairs apart, leading to notable advancements in HSI clustering performance [33–38]. Existing contrastive learning-based HSI clustering methods can be divided into two main groups based on their use of data augmentation. This first category, known as augmentation-dependent methods. These techniques apply transformations such as rotation, cropping, or noise injection to create augmented samples [33, 34]. However, such modifications risk distorting the inherent structure of HSI data, possibly shifting the semantic meaning of the

Y. Ding et al., *Graph Neural Network for Hyperspectral Image Clustering*, Intelligent Perception and Information Processing, https://doi.org/10.1007/978-981-96-7710-8_2

samples. In another line of research, the second category, knowns as augmentation-free methods. Instead of artificial augmentations, these approaches designate the k-nearest neighbors of each sample as positives while treating all others as negatives [35, 36]. A key drawback, however, is that the selected positives may not always be accurate, which can destabilize model training. Given these challenges, there is a pressing need for a robust augmentation strategy that overcomes the limitations of both existing paradigms while preserving data integrity and improving clustering reliability.

A critical limitation persists in current contrastive clustering methods for HSI analysis. While data augmentation may induce semantic shifts, most contrastive learning frameworks naively assume uniform sample contributions to the learning objective. This uniform optimization approach results in two key issues: (i) network training becomes disproportionately driven by easily separable samples, marginalizing more challenging but informative instances, and (ii) the model remains vulnerable to noise from unlabeled background regions. Existing hard sample mining techniques from conventional image processing prove inadequate for HSI applications, as they fail to account for the unique interplay between spectral signatures and spatial consistency. Consider Fig. 2.1, where inter-class samples (e.g., pair 3) may demonstrate spectral similarity, while intra-class samples (e.g., pair 4) could show substantial spectral variance due to temporal changes. The unsupervised nature of HSI clustering is further complicated by ambiguous background pixels that introduce noise and degrade clustering performance. Notably, Fig. 2.2 reveals that prevailing contrastive learning methods employ an indiscriminate treatment of all samples. This uniform optimization strategy creates a training bias where straightforward samples dominate the learning process, while critical boundary samples that define cluster separation receive insufficient attention [39]. Such oversight significantly compromises the model's ability to learn discriminative features for challenging cases.

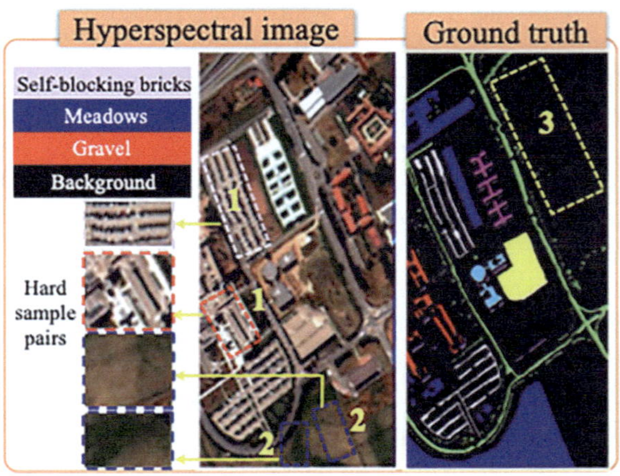

Fig. 2.1 In hyperspectral imagery, hard samples can be classified into three types: (i) hard positive sample pairs, which belong to the same cluster but exhibit low similarity, such as pair 1; (ii) hard negative sample pairs, which belong to different clusters but display high similarity, such as pair 2; (iii) these are ambiguous background pixels that are challenging to classify and may disrupt neighboring samples, samples 3

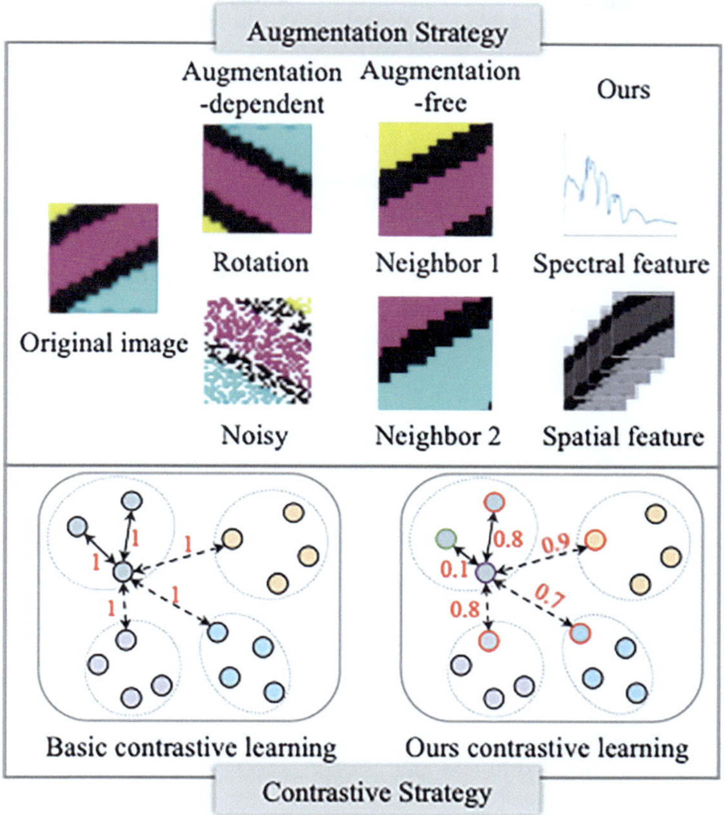

Fig. 2.2 Our method introduces two key innovations that distinguish it from conventional approaches: (i) Augmentation strategy: While existing methods either rely on artificial perturbations (e.g., noise injection) or simple neighbor selection for view generation, our technique develops a sophisticated dual-view construction mechanism that comprehensively integrates both spatial contextual patterns and spectral signatures, enabling more robust feature representation learning through multi-perspective analysis; (ii) Contrastive strategy: Departing from the naive uniform treatment paradigm adopted by current techniques, we implement an adaptive weighting scheme that dynamically recalibrates sample importance during contrastive optimization, thereby mitigating the prevalent bias toward trivial samples while simultaneously enhancing focus on discriminative boundary cases and hard samples that are crucial for precise clustering performance, ultimately yielding more balanced and representative feature embeddings

To address these limitations, we propose Spatial-Spectral Graph Contrastive Clustering with Hard Sample Mining (SSGCC), a novel framework that systematically leverages spatial-spectral information to identify and prioritize hard samples while avoiding the noise issues associated with conventional data augmentation. Our approach centers on superpixel anchors, using their spatial and spectral features as dual-branch inputs to graph autoencoders, which enables robust feature learning without artificial perturbations. By introducing clustering-oriented consistency learning, we enforce agreement between spatial and spectral embeddings, enhancing the semantic quality of the learned representations. Furthermore, we develop an adaptive contrastive learning mechanism that first identifies high-confidence samples through cross-domain consensus, then employs a dynamic weight modulation strategy to selectively emphasize challenging cases—specifically focusing on positive pairs with low similarity and negative pairs with high similarity. This integrated approach not only overcomes the limitations of uniform sample treatment but also effectively handles the unique challenges of HSI data, including spectral variability and spatial complexity, resulting in more discriminative and reliable clustering performance.

In summary, our work presents three fundamental contributions to hyperspectral image clustering:

(1) We introduce SSGCC as the first HSI clustering framework to systematically incorporate hard sample mining, addressing a critical gap in existing approaches.
(2) We develop an innovative spatial-spectral view construction method utilizing superpixel segmentation, complemented by a novel consistency loss function that effectively aligns clustering results across both spatial and spectral domains.
(3) We pioneer a contrastive learning strategy that specifically targets hard samples through integrated spatial-spectral feature analysis, significantly enhancing representation learning for challenging cases.
(4) Comprehensive experimental validation across four benchmark HSI datasets consistently demonstrates our method's superior performance, establishing new state-of-the-art results while confirming the practical viability of our technical innovations in real-world HSI analysis scenarios.

2.2 Related Work

2.2.1 Deep Clustering for Large-Scale HSI

Hyperspectral image clustering seeks to automatically group pixels into meaningful categories through unsupervised feature learning [1, 40–42]. Current approaches can be categorized based on dataset scale: small-scale methods [38, 43] handle limited samples from specialized scenarios, while large-scale techniques [26, 35, 44] address more complex, realistic conditions that demand greater computational resources. While deep learning models struggle with large-scale HSI due to their intensive computational requirements, superpixel-based alternatives have emerged as efficient solutions by exploiting the inherent homogeneity of hyperspectral data [45, 46]. These methods first partition images into irregular superpixel regions before further processing. Notable advancements include Cai et al.'s [35] superpixel pooling autoencoder for compact subspace learning and Huang et al.'s [47] hierarchical approach integrating multi-level semantic information. Graph convolutional networks have particularly advanced the field, with Zhang et al.'s [26] dual graph autoencoder (DGAE) simultaneously processing superpixel and band similarity graphs, and Ding et al.'s [48] self-correlated learning enhanced GCN. However, these methods often underutilize spatial information by employing simplistic spectral averaging within superpixels, leaving room for improved feature extraction techniques that better preserve spatial-spectral relationships.

2.2.2 *Contrastive Learning in HSI Processing*

Recent advances in unsupervised learning have witnessed the growing prominence of contrastive learning techniques [49–54], which eliminate the need for labor-intensive manual annotations. At its core, contrastive learning operates by maximizing agreement between positive sample pairs while minimizing similarity with negative pairs in the learned feature space. This discriminative approach enhances representation learning by pulling semantically similar instances closer together while pushing dissimilar ones apart in the embedding space. The effectiveness of this paradigm is mathematically formalized through the InfoNCE loss function [55], defined as:

$$l = -\log \frac{\exp(\text{sim}(z_i, z_j))}{\exp(\text{sim}(z_i, z_j)) + \sum_{k \neq j} \exp(\text{sim}(z_i, z_k))}, \tag{2.1}$$

where $\text{sim}(\cdot)$ denotes the cosine similarity. z_j and z_k form positive sample pairs and negative sample pairs with z_i respectively.

Contrastive learning has emerged as a pivotal approach for unsupervised HSI clustering [56–59], with several notable methodological advancements demonstrating its potential. Previous works have explored various contrastive strategies: Hu et al. [34] established contrastive pairs using pixel patches and their noise-augmented variants, while CMSCGC [38] generated multi-view representations by extracting complementary features like texture information to enhance positive sample alignment. Alternative approaches include Qi et al.'s [60] superpixel-level contrastive framework employing dual data augmentations (pixel sampling and model weight perturbation), and Cai et al.'s [35] neighborhood contrastive subspace clustering (NCSC) that substitutes augmentation with nearest-neighbor positive sample selection. Guan et al. [36] further advanced the field by integrating pixel-superpixel contrastive learning with pseudo-label refinement. However, these methods share a critical limitation - their uniform treatment of all samples in the contrastive objective fails to account for varying sample difficulties, ultimately constraining their discriminative power. Our work addresses this fundamental gap by introducing a novel spatial-spectral aware contrastive learning paradigm that specifically identifies and emphasizes hard samples through adaptive feature weighting, enabling more effective representation learning for challenging cases that typically determine clustering performance boundaries. Key Advantages of Our Approach: (i) Differentiated Sample Treatment: Moves beyond uniform contrastive weighting; (ii)

Spatial-Spectral Synergy: Jointly leverages both feature modalities; (iii) Boundary Sensitivity: Prioritizes discriminative hard samples; (iv) Architecture Compatibility: Integrates with existing contrastive frameworks.

2.2.3 *Hard Sample Mining in Contrastive Learning*

Hard sample mining in contrastive learning aims to identify and specially process challenging samples that are crucial for refining decision boundaries, an approach that has shown remarkable success in both image and graph domains [61–64]. Recent developments include Zhang et al.'s dual-temperature mechanism [65] for independently controlling hardness-aware properties and ProGCL's sophisticated hardness metric [66] combining similarity measures with probability estimation. Graph-based approaches have particularly advanced the field, with Tu et al.'s mutual information-based hierarchical method [39] and Liu et al.'s attribute-structure aware network [62] demonstrating impressive results. However, these existing techniques prove inadequate for hyperspectral imagery due to HSI's unique characteristics where conventional hardness measures fail to capture the domain-specific challenges arising from spectral distortions caused by seasonal variations and building reflections, along with pervasive background interference that contaminates feature extraction. To address these limitations, we develop a novel spatial-spectral hard sample mining strategy that synergistically combines both feature modalities through a dynamic weighting mechanism, enabling our model to automatically identify and emphasize truly challenging samples—particularly those with spectral ambiguities or spatial boundary complexities—while reducing attention to simpler cases, thereby significantly improving discriminative capability in HSI clustering tasks by focusing learning efforts on the most informative and difficult samples that ultimately determine clustering performance boundaries.

2.3 Methods

Our proposed Spatial-Spectral Graph Contrastive Clustering (SSGCC) framework comprises three key technical innovations designed to address the unique challenges of HSI clustering, as visually presented in Fig. 2.3. The first component establishes robust feature anchors through superpixel-guided segmentation and subsequent spatial-spectral feature extraction using an advanced graph encoder architecture, which preserves both local geometric structures and global spectral patterns. The second component introduces a novel clustering-oriented consistency learning mechanism that enforces semantic alignment between spatial and spectral feature representations, significantly enhancing the discriminative power of learned embeddings. The third and most distinctive component develops an adaptive contrastive

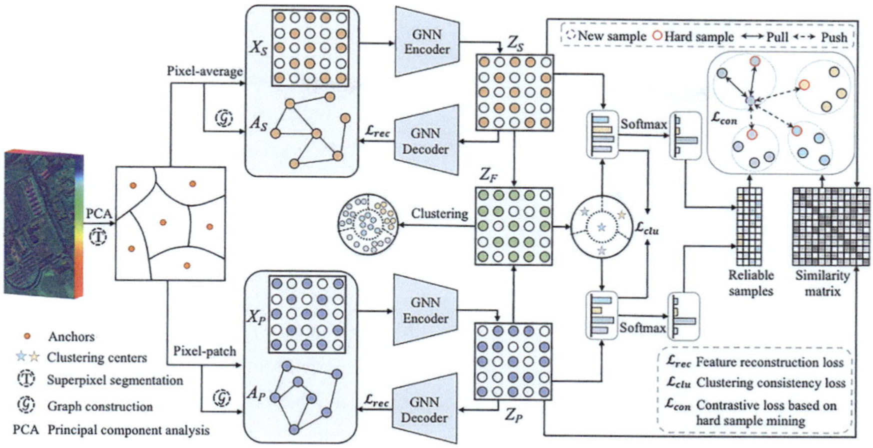

Fig. 2.3 The SSGCC framework operates through three sequential processing stages, as illustrated in Figure X. The architecture begins by identifying stable reference points through superpixel analysis, followed by comprehensive feature extraction using graph-based autoencoders that capture both geometric and spectral characteristics. Building upon these encoded representations, the system implements a novel cluster-alignment mechanism that enforces agreement between spatial and spectral similarity patterns, thereby enhancing feature discriminability. The final stage incorporates an adaptive weighting scheme within the contrastive learning process, which automatically identifies and prioritizes diagnostically challenging samples while reducing emphasis on simpler cases

learning algorithm incorporating intelligent hard sample mining, which dynamically identifies and emphasizes challenging cases during the optimization process.

2.3.1 *Notations and Definitions*

Notations. Consider a hyperspectral image represented as a three-dimensional tensor $\mathbf{X} \in \mathbb{R}^{W \times H \times D}$, containing $N = W \times H$ pixels with D spectral bands each. This data structure can be modeled as an undirected graph $\mathcal{G} = (\mathbf{X}, \mathbf{A})$, where $\mathbf{A} \in \mathbb{R}^{N \times N}$ represents the adjacency matrix encoding pairwise sample similarities through binary edge connections ($a_{ij} = 1$ if nodes v_i and v_j are connected, 0 otherwise). The normalized adjacency matrix is computed as $\tilde{\mathbf{A}} = \hat{\mathbf{D}}^{-1/2}\hat{\mathbf{A}}\hat{\mathbf{D}}^{-1/2}$, where I denotes the identity matrix and D corresponds to the diagonal degree matrix. This normalization scheme incorporates self-connections through the identity matrix while maintaining proper scaling via the degree matrix. For reference, all mathematical notations employed throughout our formulation are systematically organized in Table 2.1.

GCN. Unlike convolutional neural networks that process localized receptive fields, graph convolutional networks employ a fundamentally different paradigm by explicitly aggregating information from neighboring nodes to model long-range spatial

Table 2.1 Summary of notations

Notation	Description
$\mathcal{S}$	The set of superpixels
M	The number of superpixels
w	The patch size of anchors
K	The number of clusters
k	The number of neighbors
D^S	The dimension of X^S
$\hat{d}^S$	The dimension of Z^S
D^P	The dimension of X^P
$\hat{d}^P$	The dimension of Z^P
$N = W \times H$	The number of data points
$\mathbf{X} \in \mathbb{R}^{W \times H \times D}$	HSI cube
$\mathbf{X}^S \in \mathbb{R}^{M \times D^S}$	The spectral data matrix
$\mathbf{X}^P \in \mathbb{R}^{M \times D^P}$	The spatial data matrix
$\mathbf{A}^S \in \mathbb{R}^{M \times M}$	The adjacency matrix of spectral data
$\mathbf{A}^P \in \mathbb{R}^{M \times M}$	The adjacency matrix of spatial data
$\mathbf{Z}^S \in \mathbb{R}^{M \times d^S}$	The spectral feature matrix
$\mathbf{Z}^P \in \mathbb{R}^{M \times d^P}$	The spatial feature matrix
$\boldsymbol{\mu} \in \mathbb{R}^{K \times \hat{d}}$	The cluster center matrix
$\mathbf{P} \in \mathbb{R}^{M}$	The clustering pseudo labels
$\mathbf{Q} \in \mathbb{R}^{M \times M}$	The cluster pseudo label matrix
$\mathbf{Y} \in \mathbb{R}^{\overline{M}}$	The set of reliable samples
$\mathcal{H}$	The similarity function
$\mathcal{M}$	The weight adjustment function
$\odot$	The Hadamard product
$\mathcal{F}$	Graph encoder
$\mathcal{D}$	Graph decoder
$\Theta_{\mathcal{F}}$	The parameters of graph encoder
$\Theta_{\mathcal{D}}$	The parameters of graph decoder
$\Vert\cdot\Vert_2$	L-2 norm
$\Vert\cdot\Vert_F$	Frobenius norm

dependencies and extract discriminative features. The core computational mechanism of a GCN layer can be mathematically expressed through the following propagation rule:

$$\mathbf{Z}^{(l+1)} = \sigma\left(\mathbf{S}\mathbf{Z}^{(l)}\mathbf{W}^{(l)}\right), \tag{2.2}$$

where $\mathbf{Z}^{(0)}$ is the initial data, $\mathbf{Z}^{(l)}$ is the learned feature and l is the layer of GCN. $\mathbf{W}^{(l)}$ is the trainable weight matrix of GCN and $\sigma(\cdot)$ is an activation function.

HSI Clustering. HSI clustering aims to learn a mapping function $f : \mathbf{X} \mapsto \mathbf{Z} \in \mathbb{R}^{N\times d}$ for grouping each pixel into K distinct clusters without relying on labels, where d is the number of dimension of the latent features. In an optimally clustered outcome, the expectation is that pixels belonging to the same class should be as clustered together as possible, ensuring each cluster remains compact and distinctly segregated from other clusters.

2.3.2 *Spatial and Spectral Graph Construction*

Hyperspectral imagery presents substantial computational challenges due to its high-dimensional data structure, characterized by both spatial and spectral complexity. To address these challenges, our framework implements two key preprocessing strategies: spectral dimensionality reduction and spatial aggregation. For spectral compression, we employ principal component analysis [67] to eliminate redundant band information while preserving the most discriminative features, effectively reducing the spectral dimension from hundreds of bands to a compact yet informative representation. Simultaneously, we leverage the inherent spatial homogeneity of HSI [35] through superpixel segmentation, which groups spectrally similar adjacent pixels into homogeneous regions. In this study, we use the efficient SLIC segmentation [68] method to generate superpixels with adaptive shape and size denoted as $\mathcal{S} = \cup_{i=1}^{M} \mathbf{x}_i^{sp}$ where $M \ll N$ is the number of superpixels and $\mathbf{x}_i^{sp}$ is the i-th superpixels. Our methodology strategically selects the central pixels of superpixels as anchor points, capitalizing on their inherent spectral-spatial representativeness within each segmented region. These centroid pixels exhibit optimal homogeneity with neighboring pixels in their superpixel, making them ideal reference points that comprehensively capture regional characteristics. This anchor selection strategy offers two significant advantages over conventional approaches: (i) it preserves maximum spatial-spectral information content by leveraging the most representative points in each homogeneous region, and (ii) it eliminates the need for artificial data augmentation that typically introduces noise and semantic distortions.

Spectral feature: Since all pixels in a superpixel belong to the same class and share comparable spectral characteristics, the anchor's spectral feature is represented by averaging the spectral values of its constituent pixels. Assume that $\mathbf{X}^S \in \mathbb{R}^{M\times D^S}$ represent the spectral feature of anchors, they can be determined by

$$\mathbf{x}_i^S = \frac{\sum_{j=1}^{n_i} \mathbf{x}_j^i}{n_i}, \mathbf{x}_j^i \in \mathcal{S}_i, \tag{2.3}$$

where n_i is the number of pixels in the i-th superpixel and $\mathbf{x}_i^S \in \mathbb{R}^{1\times D^S}$ represent the spectral feature of each anchor.

Spatial feature: To integrate spatial context, we encode data points using three-dimensional local patches. This approach involves defining each point by its central spatial pixel and the adjacent pixels within a $w \times w$ window. After flatten, the spatial features of anchors can represent as $\mathbf{X}^P \in \mathbb{R}^{M\times D^P}$.

Spatial-spectral Graph Construction: GCN requires an adjacency matrix as input, so we capture the nearest samples of each anchor as neighbors and construct edges for them, with element $\mathbf{A}_{ij}$ defined as follows:

$$\mathbf{A}_{ij} = \begin{cases} 1, & \text{if } \mathbf{x}_j \in \Gamma(\mathbf{x}_i), \\ 0, & \text{otherwise}, \end{cases} \tag{2.4}$$

where $\Gamma(\cdot)$ represents the top k nearest samples set of sample. By inputting spatial features and spectral features respectively, we can obtain two adjacency matrices $\mathbf{A}^S$ and $\mathbf{A}^P \in \mathbb{R}^{M\times M}$.

2.3.3 Graph Autoencoder Module

To fully explore the topology of the constructed graph and aggregate features from neighboring nodes, we deploy two graph encoders $\mathbf{Z}^S$ and $\mathbf{Z}^P$ to caputer features. In practice, we employ a multi-layer Graph Convolutional Network (GCN) as our graph encoder. This framework iteratively refines node embeddings by propagating features across the graph structure. The process can be formally described as follows:

$$\mathbf{Z}^S = \mathcal{F}_S(\tilde{\mathbf{A}}^S, \mathbf{X}^S | \Theta_{\mathcal{F}_S}), \tag{2.5}$$

$$\mathbf{Z}^P = \mathcal{F}_P(\tilde{\mathbf{A}}^P, \mathbf{X}^P | \Theta_{\mathcal{F}_P}), \tag{2.6}$$

where $\Theta_{\mathcal{F}_S}$ and $\Theta_{\mathcal{F}_P}$ denotes the learnable parameters of two graph encoders. $\tilde{\mathbf{A}} \in \mathbb{R}^{M\times M}$ denotes the normalized adjacency matrix.

The graph encoder architecture leverages an improved multi-layer Graph Convolutional Network, following methodological advances from [17]. This network serves as decoder $D(\cdot)$ to recover both spatial and spectral characteristics of the input data. The feature reconstruction mechanism operates through the following formulation:

$$\hat{\mathbf{X}}^S = \mathcal{D}_S(\tilde{\mathbf{A}}^S, \mathbf{Z}^S | \Theta_{\mathcal{D}_S}), \tag{2.7}$$

$$\hat{\mathbf{X}}^P = \mathcal{D}_P(\tilde{\mathbf{A}}^P, \mathbf{Z}^P | \Theta_{\mathcal{D}_P}), \tag{2.8}$$

where $\hat{\mathbf{X}}^S$ and $\hat{\mathbf{X}}^P$ is the reconstruction features, $\Theta_{\mathcal{D}_S}$ and $\Theta_{\mathcal{D}_P}$ denote the learnable parameters of two graph encoders. Therefore, the individual-level reconstruction loss function could be defined as:

$$\mathcal{L}_{\text{rec}} = \left\|\mathbf{X}^S - \hat{\mathbf{X}}^S\right\|_F^2 + \left\|\mathbf{X}^P - \hat{\mathbf{X}}^P\right\|_F^2, \tag{2.9}$$

where $\|\cdot\|_F$ represents the Frobenius norm.

2.3.4 Cluster-Oriented Consistency Learning

To enable cross-domain knowledge transfer between spatial and spectral representations, we introduce cluster-aligned consistency learning. This framework is designed to capture intrinsic sample correlations through learned feature representations, ultimately improving unsupervised hyperspectral image clustering performance. The approach establishes semantic correspondence by measuring pairwise node similarities across dual-view embedding spaces.

In detail, we first use the attention-based weight fusion method to obtain the fused latent feature Z^F:

$$\mathbf{Z}^F = \mathbf{W}_1 \odot \mathbf{Z}^S + \mathbf{W}_2 \odot \mathbf{Z}^P, \tag{2.10}$$

where $\odot$ is the Hadamard product and $\mathbf{W}_1, \mathbf{W}_2 \in \mathbb{R}^{M \times \hat{d}}$ are trainable weight matrices to control the importance of spatial-spectral features.

More precisely, we compute the fused features $\mathbf{Z}^F$ of the dual branches and employ the K-means algorithm $\mathcal{K}(\cdot)$ to ascertain the clustering centroid of the fused feature:

$$\{\boldsymbol{\mu}, \mathbf{P}\} \leftarrow \mathcal{K}(\mathbf{Z}^F), \tag{2.11}$$

where $\boldsymbol{\mu} \in \mathbb{R}^{K \times \hat{d}}$ denotes the cluster center matrix and $\mathbf{P} \in \mathbb{R}^M$ is the clustering pseudo labels. Then we first measure the similarity between the i-th node embedding $\mathbf{z}_i$ and the k-th cluster centroid $\mathbf{c}_k$ by student's t-distribution as follows,

$$q_{ij}^S = \frac{(1 + \left\|\mathbf{z}_i^S - \boldsymbol{\mu}_j\right\|^2/\eta)^{(-\frac{\eta+1}{2})}}{\sum_j^K (1 + \left\|\mathbf{z}_i^S - \boldsymbol{\mu}_j\right\|^2/\eta)^{(-\frac{\eta+1}{2})}}, \tag{2.12}$$

$$q_{ij}^P = \frac{(1 + \|\mathbf{z}_i^P - \boldsymbol{\mu}_j\|^2/\eta)^{(-\frac{\eta+1}{2})}}{\sum_j^K (1 + \|\mathbf{z}_i^P - \boldsymbol{\mu}_j\|^2/\eta)^{(-\frac{\eta+1}{2})}}, \tag{2.13}$$

where q_{ij} refers to the probability of assigning i-th node to the j-th cluster. Here, η denotes the degrees of freedom, and we set $\eta = 1$ in all of our experiments.

Leveraging similarity distributions from both spectral and spatial domains, we enforce cross-view consistency to enable effective knowledge transfer and mutually reinforce feature representations. The consistency learning objective is formally expressed as:

$$q_{ij}^{P} = \mathcal{L}_{\text{clu}} = \frac{1}{2M} \sum_{i=1}^{M} \sum_{j=1}^{K} \left(\text{KL}\left(\mathbf{q}_{ij}^{S} \| \mathbf{q}_{ij}^{P} \right) + \text{KL}\left(\mathbf{q}_{ij}^{P} \| \mathbf{q}_{ij}^{S} \right) \right), \tag{2.14}$$

where $\text{KL}(\cdot\|\cdot)$ is the Kullback–Leibler (KL) divergence. In the training, we minimize $\mathcal{L}_{\text{clu}}$ to optimize our proposed SSGCC and enhance self-supervised learning.

Algorithm 1 Learning Procedure for SSGCC

Input: Hyperspectral data cube $\mathbf{X}$, input window size w, neighborhood parameter k, superpixel count M, ant the training iterations I.
Output: Clustering results.
Initialize the parameters of the network.
Construct superpixel set $\mathcal{S}$ by using superpixel segmentation $\mathbf{T}$.
Construct the spectral and spatial features of the anchors based on the pixel feature average and sliding window.
Construct spectral matrix $\mathbf{A}^S$ and spatial adjacency matrix $\mathbf{A}^P$ by Eq. (2.4).
for $i = 1$ to $\leq I$ **do**
Obtain $\mathbf{Z}^S$ and $\mathbf{Z}^P$ with f_S and f_P by Eqs. (2.5) and (2.6).
Obtain fused feature $\mathbf{Z}^F$ by Eq. (2.10).
Obtain pseudo labels $\mathbf{Q}$ by Eq. (2.15).
Design similarity function $\mathcal{H}$ by Eq. (2.16).
Design weight modulating function $\mathcal{M}$ by Eq. (2.17).
Calculate reconstruction loss $\mathcal{L}_{\text{rec}}$ by Eq. (2.9).
Calculate clustering consistency loss $\mathcal{L}_{\text{clu}}$ by Eq. (2.14).
Calculate hard sample mining-based contrastive loss $\mathcal{L}_{\text{con}}$ by Eq. (2.18).
Update parameters of the network by minimizing Eq. (2.19).
end for
Using K-means on fused feature $\mathbf{Z}^F$ to get the cluster result $\mathbf{P}$.
return P

Guided by the cluster consistency constraint outlined in Eq. (2.14), we identify and record those samples for which the labels predicted by the spectral and spatial branches concur as reliable samples set $\mathbf{Y} \in \mathbb{R}^{\overline{M}}$, where $\overline{M} < M$ is the number of reliable samples. Based on clustering pseudo labels $\mathbf{P}$, we calculate the sample pair pseudo labels $\mathbf{Q} \in \mathbb{R}^{M \times M}$ as follows:

$$\mathbf{Q}_{ij} = \begin{cases} 1 \ \mathbf{P}_i = \mathbf{P}_j, \\ 0 \ \mathbf{P}_i \neq \mathbf{P}_j. \end{cases} \tag{2.15}$$

Here, a value of $\mathbf{Q}_{ij} = 1$ indicates that i-th and j-th samples belong to the same cluster, suggesting they are more likely to constitute a positive sample pair. Conversely, they are most likely to represent a negative sample pair.

2.3.5 Hard Sample Mining-Based Contrastive Learning

The conventional contrastive loss formulation in Eq. (2.1) processes all samples equally, failing to account for varying difficulty levels among instances. This uniform treatment results in suboptimal feature discrimination. To address this limitation, we propose a novel hard sample mining framework that strategically utilizes: the high-confidence reference samples **Y**, cluster-assignment pseudo-labels **Q**, and the similarity metric $\mathcal{H}$ to identify and emphasize challenging instances during representation learning.

$$\mathcal{H}(\mathrm{i},\mathrm{j}) = \frac{(\mathbf{Z}_{\mathrm{i}}^{\mathrm{S}})^{\top}\mathbf{Z}_{\mathrm{j}}^{\mathrm{F}}}{2\cdot\left\|\mathbf{Z}_{\mathrm{i}}^{\mathrm{S}}\right\|\cdot\left\|\mathbf{Z}_{\mathrm{j}}^{\mathrm{F}}\right\|} + \frac{(\mathbf{Z}_{\mathrm{i}}^{\mathrm{P}})^{\top}\mathbf{Z}_{\mathrm{j}}^{\mathrm{F}}}{2\cdot\left\|\mathbf{Z}_{\mathrm{i}}^{\mathrm{P}}\right\|\cdot\left\|\mathbf{Z}_{\mathrm{j}}^{\mathrm{F}}\right\|}, \tag{2.16}$$

where $i, j \in \{1, 2, ..., M\}$. Leveraging reliable samples **Y**, cluster pseudo labels **Q**, and the similarity function $\mathcal{H}$, we have devised a weight adjustment function $\mathcal{M}$ to dynamically modulate the weights of sample pairs throughout the training process. The calculation of $\mathcal{M}$ is as follows:

$$\mathcal{M}(i,j) = \begin{cases} 1, i \notin Y \cup j \notin Y, \\ |\mathbf{Q}_{ij} - \mathrm{Norm}(H(i,j))|^{\beta}, \text{others}, \end{cases} \tag{2.17}$$

where Norm denotes the min–max normalization and $\beta \geq 1$ is a scaling factor. When not all samples exhibit high confidence ($i \notin \mathbf{Y} \cup j \notin \mathbf{Y}$), we resort to using the classic infoNCE loss function. However, in cases where all samples are of high confidence, our method is adept at dynamically adjusting weights based on the similarity and pseudo information.

Our investigation reveals the critical function of weight modulator $\mathcal{M}$ in the hard sample mining process. As demonstrated in Fig. 2.1, we operationalize hard samples through two distinct categories: (i) Intra-cluster samples exhibiting low pairwise similarity (hard positives), and (ii) Inter-cluster samples demonstrating high pairwise similarity (hard negatives). The modulation function $\mathcal{M}$ assigns higher weights to sample pairs that meet these conditions, while simpler sample pairs receive lower weights.

Consequently, $\mathcal{M}$ up-weights positive sample pairs with low similarity (the hard ones) and down-weights those with high similarity (the easy ones).

Based on $\mathcal{H}$ and $\mathcal{M}$, we formulate the hard sample mining-based contrastive loss as follows:

$$\mathcal{L}_{\mathrm{con}} = \frac{1}{M}\sum_{i,j=1}^{M} -\log\left(\frac{e^{\mathcal{M}(i,i)\cdot\mathcal{H}(i,i)}}{e^{\mathcal{M}(i,i)\cdot\mathcal{H}(i,i)} + \sum_{i\neq j} e^{\mathcal{M}(i,j)\cdot\mathcal{H}(i,j)}}\right). \tag{2.18}$$

Unlike conventional contrastive learning approaches that assign equal importance to all samples, our method introduces a novel hard sample mining strategy. By leveraging spectral-spatial cues, the network prioritizes challenging sample pairs, enhancing their influence during training. Concurrently, the weights of difficult pairs are adaptively increased, while those of simpler pairs are reduced. This dynamic weighting mechanism strengthens the model's discriminative power.

2.3.6 The Overall Loss Function

In summary, we propose a new spectral-spatial graph contrastive clustering framework incorporating hard sample mining for large-scale hyperspectral images (HSI). Throughout training, the model optimizes three key components jointly: graph encoders, a cluster consistency module, and a contrastive learning regularizer guided by hard sample mining. These elements are unified under the following objective function:

$$\mathcal{L} = \mathcal{L}_{\text{rec}} + \sigma_1 * \mathcal{L}_{\text{clu}} + \sigma_2 * \mathcal{L}_{\text{con}}, \tag{2.19}$$

where σ_1 and σ_2 are trade-off parameters. The detailed learning procedure of the proposed SSGCC is described in 0.

2.3.7 Complexity Analysis

We evaluate computational complexity from two perspectives: model architecture and loss computation. For tractability, we denote the input feature dimensionality as D, the layer-wise graph autoencoder dimensions as $d_1, \ldots, d_L$, and the latent embedding dimension as $\hat{d}$. The complexities of graph encoder is $\mathcal{O}\left(|E| \sum_{i=1}^{L} d_i d_{i-1}\right)$, where $|E|$ is the nubmer of edge. The time complexities of clustering consistency loss is $\mathcal{O}(MK\hat{d})$, where K is the nubmer of class. Finally, the time complexity of constructing $\mathcal{H}$ and $\mathcal{M}$ are $\mathcal{O}(M^2\hat{d})$. Thus, the overall complexity is $\mathcal{O}\left(|E| \sum_{i=1}^{L} d_i d_{i-1} + MK\hat{d} + M^2\hat{d}\right)$. Since $K \ll M$, the overall computational complexity is approximately $\mathcal{O}\left(|E| \sum_{i=1}^{L} d_i d_{i-1} + M^2\hat{d}\right)$ (Table 2.2).

Table 2.2 Hyper-parameter settings

Parameters		Salinas	Pavia University	Trento	Xu
Setting	M	2000	3000	1750	1000
	w	11	11	9	7
	σ_1	10	1000	1	1
	σ_2	10	1000	1	1
	β	3	3	2	2
	k	45	50	50	45
Range	M	$\{500, \ldots, 3000\}$, $\{1500, \ldots, 4000\}$, $\{500, \ldots, 1750\}$			
	w	$\{1, 3, 5, 7, 9, 11\}$			
	σ_1	$\{0.1, 1, 10, 100, 1000, 10000\}$			
	σ_2	$\{0.1, 1, 10, 100, 1000, 10000\}$			
	β	$\{1, 2, 3, 4\}$			
	k	$\{15, 20, 25, 30, 35, 40, 45, 50, 55, 60\}$			

2.4 Experiments

2.4.1 Experimental Setup

(1) Datasets: To enable rigorous evaluation of the proposed models, we employ four benchmark datasets in our experiments. Figure 2.4 presents corresponding false-color composites alongside their superpixel segmentation results for visual comparison.

Pavia University. The dataset was captured during an aerial survey conducted in Pavia, Northern Italy (2002) using the ROSIS imaging spectrometer. Following the elimination of 12 noise-corrupted bands, the refined dataset comprises 103 spectral

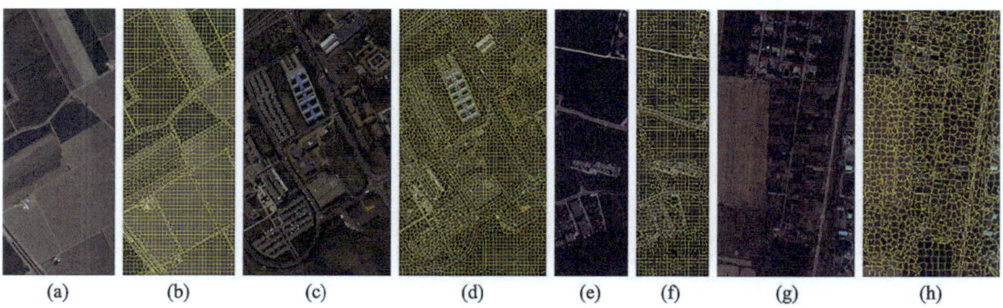

Fig. 2.4 False color images of the datasets and visualizations of superpixel segmentation. **a** False-color image of Salinas, RGB: [11, 21, 32]. **b** Segmentation of Salinas. **c** False-color image of Pavia University, RGB: [12, 41, 55]. **d** Segmentation of Pavia University. **e** False-color image of Trento, RGB: [3, 24, 60]. **f** Segmentation of Trento. **g** False-color image of XuZhou, RGB: [1, 13, 30]. **h** Segmentation of XuZhou

channels. With a spatial dimension of 610 × 340 pixels and a resolution of 1.3 m per pixel, it provides detailed coverage of urban terrain. After background removal, the processed Pavia University dataset contains 42,766 annotated samples across 19 distinct land-cover categories.

Salinas. Acquired in 1998, the original dataset contained 224 spectral channels covering wavelengths from 360 to 2500 nm. The images have a spatial resolution of 512 × 217 pixels. Following the removal of bands affected by atmospheric absorption, the final curated dataset consists of 204 spectral bands. Post-background elimination, the Salina dataset includes 54,129 annotated samples distributed across 16 distinct land-cover classes.

Trento. The Trento dataset was acquired over rural areas near Trento, Italy. This hyperspectral collection contains 63 spectral channels covering the visible to near-infrared range (420.89–989.09 nm), with a spatial extent of 600 × 166 pixels. Following background removal, the processed dataset contains 30,214 labeled samples representing six distinct land-cover categories.

XuZhou. The XuZhou dataset was acquired through airborne hyperspectral imaging using a HYSPEX sensor, focusing on peri-urban transition zones. This collection features 436 spectral channels with a spatial resolution of 500 × 260 pixels, documenting mixed urban–rural landscapes. Following preprocessing to eliminate background elements, the curated dataset contains 68,877 annotated samples categorized into nine distinct land-use classes.

(2) To demonstrate the efficacy of our Spatial-Spectral Graph Contrastive Clustering (SSGCC) approach, we perform comparative evaluations against sixteen established clustering techniques:

- **K-means (TPAMI'02)** [41]: A centroid-based unsupervised learning baseline.
- **FCM (SSBM'13)** [40]: Fuzzy C-means clustering with objective-function optimization.
- **SSC (TAPMI'13)** [69]: Classic sparse subspace clustering.
- **AEC (ICML'12)** [70]: Autoencoder-driven deep clustering.
- **DEC (ICML'16)** [71]: Joint deep feature and cluster assignment learning.
- **IDEC (IDEC'17)** [72]: Enhanced deep embedding with local-structure preservation.
- **S^5C (NeurIPS'19)** [21]: Scalable sparse clustering via selective sampling.
- **HESSC (RS'20)** [42]: Hierarchical efficient clustering for HSI.
- **MS^2A-Net (JSTARS'22)** [15]: Multiscale spectral-spatial association network.
- **DGAE (TCSVT'22)** [26]: Dual graph autoencoder (pixel- and band-level).
- **NCSC (TGRS'22)** [35]: Neighborhood contrastive subspace clustering.
- **AGCSC (CVPR'23)** [20]: Adaptive graph convolutional subspace clustering.

- **DSCRLE (TGRS'23)** [14]: Deep spectral clustering with regularized embedding.
- **PSCPC (ICASSP'24)** [36]: Pixel-superpixel contrastive learning with pseudo-label refinement.
- **CMSCGC (TGRS'24)** [38]: Multi-view contrastive clustering for HSI.
- **SDST (TGRS'24)** [44]: Self-supervised double-structure transformer.

(3) To facilitate a fair evaluation of the proposed SSGCC against baseline models, we perform ten repeated trials under consistent experimental settings, leveraging a 24GB RTX 3090 GPU and 64GB memory. The critical hyperparameters of SSGCC are outlined in Table 2.4. All methods undergo 100 training epochs across ten independent executions. The learning rate and weight decay are configured at 1×10^{-3} and 5×10^{-4}, respectively, with optimization handled by the Adam algorithm. For graph encoding and decoding, a three-layer Graph Convolutional Network (GCN) is adopted, featuring hidden and output layer dimensions of 128, 256, and 512. Baseline models utilize their optimal parameters, as documented in the referenced chapter, along with publicly available implementations, to ensure reproducibility. Notably, due to scalability constraints in AGCSC and CMSCGC when processing large datasets, we integrate a preprocessing stage that incorporates superpixel-based inputs.

To rigorously assess model performance, we adopt four widely recognized metrics: overall accuracy (ACC), Kappa coefficient, normalized mutual information (NMI), and adjusted Rand index (ARI) [73–80]. Among these, ACC and NMI are bounded within [0, 1], whereas Kappa and ARI can assume values in the interval [−1, 1], reflecting varying degrees of agreement and clustering quality.

2.4.2 Experimental Results

To evaluate the effectiveness of our approach, we conduct a comparative analysis between the proposed SSGCC and state-of-the-art hyperspectral image (HSI) clustering methods. The quantitative results, presented in Table 2.3, reveal several important findings:

(1) The SSGCC framework demonstrates superior performance across all evaluated benchmarks, attaining optimal results in all four key metrics. This notable advancement underscores the efficacy of its spatial-spectral graph architecture and contrastive learning strategy, which effectively identifies challenging sample pairs and dynamically optimizes their influence during training.
(2) Modern contrastive clustering techniques have demonstrated significant advantages over traditional graph-based methods, primarily due to their capacity for extracting richer semantic structures from data. Unlike conventional approaches, contrastive learning frameworks learn more discriminative representations through structured optimization, thereby improving clustering efficacy. A key

Table 2.3 The clustering results on four HSI datasets

No	Salinas				Pavia University				Trento				XuZhou			
	ACC	Kappa	NMI	ARI	ACC	Kappa	NMI	ARI	ACC	Kappa	NMI	ARI	ACC	Kappa	NMI	ARI
K-means	61.11	57.58	71.24	48.20	51.74	41.99	52.14	31.17	62.81	52.96	46.18	34.26	40.42	29.58	42.40	26.60
FCM	55.98	52.26	68.77	43.65	42.73	33.79	49.95	31.17	50.68	41.27	46.18	28.00	39.91	31.32	42.24	24.87
SSC	65.46	62.34	76.47	58.02	52.04	41.57	42.13	33.46	76.59	69.65	66.92	71.70	69.74	63.23	57.58	57.88
AEC	63.54	59.32	76.77	57.62	45.75	35.25	51.76	32.41	77.56	70.85	77.20	79.84	66.66	59.09	64.97	65.96
DEC	57.22	51.46	72.78	54.52	45.14	35.22	54.01	28.82	64.88	53.66	66.00	58.50	49.65	37.34	42.40	36.66
IDEC	62.21	57.91	75.50	55.45	44.79	32.95	48.48	32.34	72.99	66.03	78.57	74.93	67.75	60.35	65.84	67.90
S^5C	53.51	49.34	62.08	39.52	48.36	37.73	43.23	25.08	47.42	32.19	38.68	23.70	63.14	55.04	52.26	51.57
HESSC	52.93	47.87	60.03	41.50	47.71	36.26	49.43	29.27	49.94	30.31	32.83	21.92	42.35	26.69	32.42	25.49
MS^2A-Net	64.63	60.31	74.47	59.95	60.40	48.15	53.36	44.77	83.60	78.14	76.24	81.28	62.61	53.77	58.21	55.28
DGAE	59.50	55.60	70.89	47.87	52.65	42.89	47.55	31.93	79.85	73.00	65.88	70.65	67.61	59.93	61.05	61.36
NCSC	74.97	72.07	79.69	66.51	51.07	42.11	45.31	32.81	66.85	58.23	63.07	58.06	74.03	68.33	72.39	67.95
AGCSC	63.84	59.78	76.65	55.91	57.63	46.99	47.60	36.57	65.52	56.63	59.13	53.91	76.07	70.39	69.52	67.77
DSCRLE	57.13	52.89	60.86	35.94	48.50	36.54	44.92	22.68	77.11	69.04	65.69	70.31	71.06	64.96	62.28	56.74
PSCPC	65.19	60.21	61.08	65.53	59.36	45.16	50.44	58.41	78.26	82.44	74.35	74.70	74.14	67.86	68.48	73.03
CMSCGC	72.16	66.29	69.16	77.93	57.93	43.46	49.19	57.57	84.77	81.90	79.88	84.81	72.06	66.62	66.01	72.36
SDST	74.33	71.30	80.11	61.86	50.70	39.17	42.66	29.19	82.96	76.55	71.92	74.90	67.00	57.72	62.82	60.15
Ours	**81.99**	**76.36**	**80.30**	**86.21**	**63.74**	**52.86**	**54.88**	**59.27**	**91.62**	**93.57**	**88.77**	**87.80**	**80.74**	**74.92**	**76.29**	**77.93**

The best and suboptimal results are highlighted with **bold** and underline, respectively

Table 2.4 Running time (second) of deep learning-based methods on four datasets

Dataset	AE	DEC	IDEC	HESSC	MS^2A-Net	DGAE	NCSC	DSCRLE	PSCPC	CMSCGC	SDST	Ours
Salinas	949	794	586	730	488	46	500	125	92	622	986	58
Pavia University	824	647	373	1014	152	43	621	235	190	735	925	116
Trento	524	443	190	555	106	39	435	124	86	831	552	36
XuZhou	1113	950	754	960	473	117	420	538	101	573	1842	39

strength of our SSGCC method is its proficiency in detecting challenging samples, which further elevates its performance beyond standard contrastive techniques. Empirical results highlight SSGCC's substantial improvements over NCSC and CMSCGC, with absolute accuracy (ACC) increases of 7.02%/9.83%, 12.67%/5.81%, 24.77%/6.85%, and 6.71%/8.68% across four benchmark datasets.

(3) Graph convolutional networks demonstrate superior performance compared to traditional techniques by effectively aggregating local node features. Among clustering algorithms, AGCSC substantially improves upon classical approaches such as K-means and SSC through its adaptive neighborhood feature integration. In deep learning-based clustering, our proposed SSGCC framework achieves notable gains over both convolutional (PSCPC) and transformer architectures (SDST). Quantitative evaluations reveal consistent accuracy improvements of 16.8%/7.66%, 4.38%/13.04%, 13.36%/8.66%, and 6.6%/13.74% across benchmark datasets, demonstrating SSGCC's robust performance advantages.

2.4.3 *Qualitative Comparison*

The clustering results visualized in Figs. 2.5, 2.6, 2.7 and 2.8 demonstrate the superior performance of SSGCC compared to baseline models across all four datasets. Our approach generates more distinct cluster separations and sharper boundaries, particularly evident in complex classification scenarios. For instance, on the Salinas dataset, SSGCC successfully discriminates between the four romaine lettuce varieties that other methods consistently misclassify. The Trento dataset results (Fig. 2.7) further highlight this advantage, where our model accurately separates vineyard and woodland areas while competing algorithms produce blurred transitional regions and classification errors. This enhanced capability stems from SSGCC's innovative focus on difficult-to-classify samples, which substantially improves classification robustness by minimizing boundary ambiguities.

To further validate the effectiveness of SSGCC, Fig. 2.9 presents T-SNE visualizations of the learned embedding distributions. These visualizations reveal several key advantages of our approach: (i) enhanced inter-cluster separation with more distinct boundaries, (ii) tighter intra-cluster cohesion while maintaining appropriate diversity, and (iii) significantly greater margin distances between different categories. These characteristics collectively demonstrate SSGCC's superior capacity for generating highly discriminative feature representations compared to baseline methods.

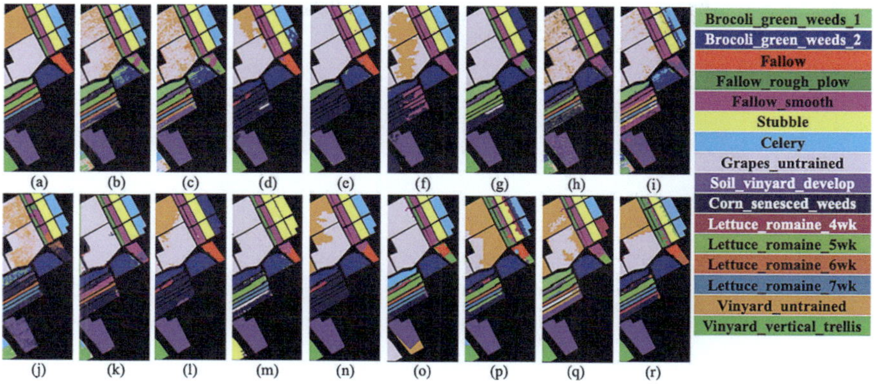

Fig. 2.5 Clustering maps on Salinas dataset. **a** ground truth; **b** K-means; **c** FCM; **d** SSC; **e** AE; **f** DEC; **g** IDEC; **h** S^5C; **i** HESSC; **j** MS^2A-Net; **k** DGAE; **l** NCSC; **m** AGCSC; **n** DSCRLE; **o** PSCPC; **p** CMSCGC; **q** SDST; **r** Our proposed SSGCC

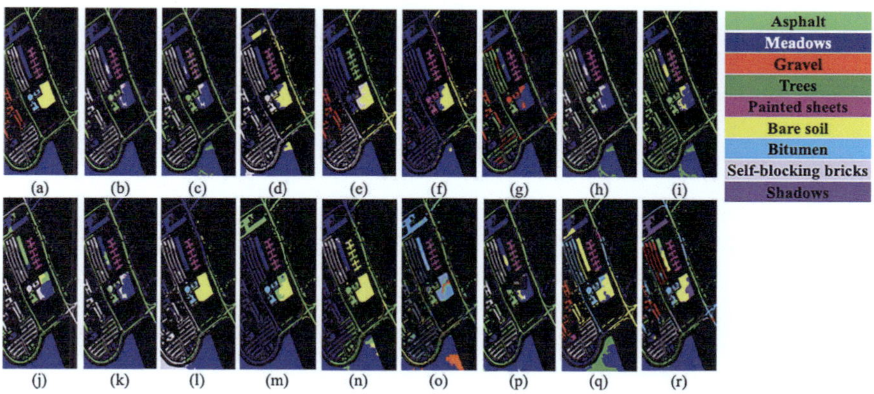

Fig. 2.6 Clustering maps on Pavia University dataset. **a** ground truth; **b** K-means; **c** FCM; **d** SSC; **e** AE; **f** DEC; **g** IDEC; **h** S^5C; **i** HESSC; **j** MS^2A-Net; **k** DGAE; **l** NCSC; **m** AGCSC; **n** DSCRLE; **o** PSCPC; **p** CMSCGC; **q** SDST; **r** Our proposed SSGCC

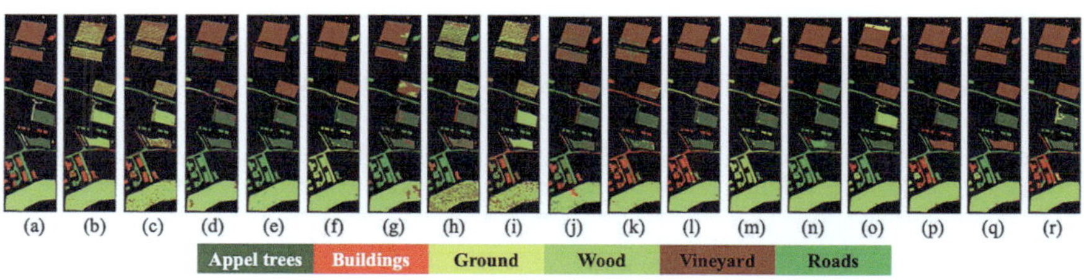

Fig. 2.7 Clustering maps on Trento dataset. **a** ground truth; **b** K-means; **c** FCM; **d** SSC; **e** AE; **f** DEC; **g** IDEC; **h** S^5C; **i** HESSC; **j** MS^2A-Net; **k** DGAE; **l** NCSC; **m** AGCSC; **n** DSCRLE; **o** PSCPC; **p** CMSCGC; **q** SDST; **r** Our proposed SSGCC

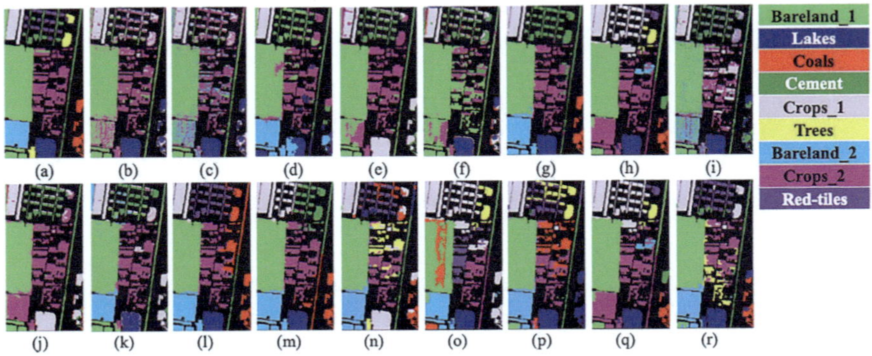

Fig. 2.8 Clustering maps on XuZhou dataset. **a** ground truth; **b** K-means; **c** FCM; **d** SSC; **e** AE; **f** DEC; **g** IDEC; **h** S^5C; **i** HESSC; **j** MS^2A-Net; **k** DGAE; **l** NCSC; **m** AGCSC; **n** DSCRLE; **o** PSCPC; **p** CMSCGC; **q** SDST; **r** Our proposed SSGCC

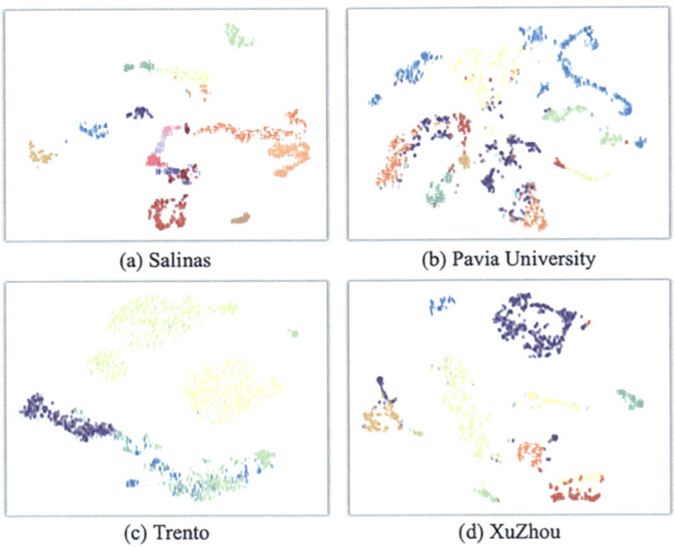

Fig. 2.9 T-SNE Visualization of the proposed SSGCC on the four datasets

2.4.4 Running Time

To evaluate computational efficiency, we conducted runtime comparisons between SSGCC and existing deep learning-based HSI clustering methods across four benchmark datasets. As evidenced in Table 2.4, our approach achieves markedly faster processing speeds. Traditional techniques like AE, DEC, and IDEC demonstrate slower performance due to their pixel-wise processing requirements and batch-based data loading mechanisms. Although NCSC and CMSCGC employ superpixel preprocessing, their reliance on subspace clustering introduces iterative optimization procedures that are computationally intensive ($\mathcal{O}(N^3)$ complexity), despite improving result accuracy. The SDST method, while effective at handling spatial correlations in large datasets, similarly suffers from high computational overhead. SSGCC's superior efficiency stems from its carefully designed architecture that optimally balances computational demands with clustering performance.

2.4.5 Ablation Study

To systematically evaluate the impact of key components in our framework, we perform ablation studies focusing on three critical aspects: (i) the primary loss function, (ii) data augmentation techniques, and (iii) contrastive learning mechanisms. Through controlled experiments where we alternately remove individual components or modify augmentation approaches, we quantitatively assess their relative importance and effects on model performance. The comprehensive results of these experiments are presented in Table 2.5, providing clear insights into each component's contribution to the overall system effectiveness.

(1) *Ablation on the Main Loss*: We define w/o $\mathcal{L}_{\text{rec}}$, w/o $\mathcal{L}_{\text{clu}}$ and w/o $\mathcal{L}_{\text{con}}$ as the proposed SSGCC variants without reconstruction loss, clustering consistent loss and hard sample mining based contrastive learning loss, respectively. The results indicated that the MCGC method exhibited the best performance. When removing the clustering consistency loss and contrast loss, the accuracy of the model drops by 1.54%/8.24%, 1.22%/9.72, 2.85%/10.32%, and 2.82%/5.16% on the four datasets respectively. This indicates that each module of the network is effective and their absence could result in performance degradation.
(2) *Ablation on the Augmentation strategy*: To prevent noise artifacts from conventional augmentation approaches, we construct dual views using extracted spatial-spectral features. We evaluate SSGCC against standard augmentation methods including feature masking (random 30% feature removal), feature noising (random 30% edge addition), and edge perturbation (random 30% edge modification). Experimental results demonstrate consistent accuracy reductions of 2%-6% for these traditional methods, confirming they introduce semantic noise and feature distortion. This outcome highlights the advantage of our spatial-spectral feature extraction method for robust contrastive learning.
(3) *Ablation on the Contrastive Scheme*: To demonstrate the effectiveness of our proposed contrastive learning method based on hard sample mining, we compare the basic contrastive learning (w/o $\mathcal{M}$) with our proposed SSGCC. From the results, we can observe that compared with the baseline, our contrastive learning strategy has increased by 3.6%, 4.07%, 3.32% and 2.51% respectively. This shows that our dynamic weight strategy can effectively mine hard samples and improve the model's discriminative ability.

Table 2.5 Ablation experiments on SSGCC in three aspects: main loss, augmentation strategy and contrastive scheme

Dataset	Metric	Main loss			Augmentation strategy			Contrastive scheme	
		w/o $\mathcal{L}_{rec}$	w/o $\mathcal{L}_{clu}$	w/o $\mathcal{L}_{con}$	Feature mask	Feature noise	Edge permutation	w/o $\mathcal{M}$	Ours
Salinas	ACC	71.28 ± 3.64	80.45 ± 0.65	73.75 ± 2.55	75.83 ± 2.92	76.87 ± 2.76	76.29 ± 2.34	78.39 ± 0.98	81.99 ± 0.84
	NMI	68.17 ± 4.07	78.65 ± 0.70	71.41 ± 2.68	73.53 ± 3.08	74.61 ± 2.98	74.17 ± 2.48	76.30 ± 1.06	80.30 ± 0.93
	ARI	77.36 ± 1.75	86.83 ± 0.56	80.61 ± 1.18	81.52 ± 1.27	82.08 ± 1.27	82.98 ± 0.96	84.83 ± 0.81	86.21 ± 1.08
	Kappa	64.87 ± 6.82	76.76 ± 0.89	71.42 ± 4.50	72.55 ± 4.85	75.45 ± 5.04	73.44 ± 2.78	73.57 ± 2.22	76.36 ± 3.20
PaviaU	ACC	51.15 ± 7.48	62.52 ± 1.33	54.02 ± 6.94	56.28 ± 3.56	58.55 ± 3.82	59.40 ± 2.63	59.66 ± 4.66	63.74 ± 1.36
	NMI	42.28 ± 7.10	52.34 ± 2.31	44.77 ± 6.76	47.42 ± 3.56	49.29 ± 3.87	49.70 ± 2.92	50.69 ± 4.83	54.88 ± 1.72
	ARI	49.42 ± 4.21	56.67 ± 2.05	52.25 ± 3.09	52.68 ± 3.32	54.64 ± 2.89	54.84 ± 2.25	56.45 ± 5.18	59.27 ± 1.78
	Kappa	39.0 ± 10.95	52.07 ± 5.32	44.49 ± 9.52	45.91 ± 7.63	45.71 ± 7.59	47.78 ± 4.64	46.26 ± 9.59	52.86 ± 1.93
Trento	ACC	77.36 ± 0.25	88.77 ± 0.93	81.30 ± 0.37	84.76 ± 0.85	86.90 ± 0.82	84.44 ± 4.27	87.85 ± 1.46	91.62 ± 0.88
	NMI	73.30 ± 0.32	85.04 ± 1.16	78.37 ± 0.50	81.08 ± 1.12	83.25 ± 1.10	79.72 ± 5.29	83.86 ± 1.91	88.77 ± 1.15
	ARI	72.78 ± 0.45	84.12 ± 0.86	76.60 ± 0.80	80.16 ± 0.96	82.83 ± 0.72	81.71 ± 2.02	82.77 ± 1.34	87.80 ± 0.97
	Kappa	77.39 ± 0.49	90.72 ± 2.07	82.75 ± 0.65	84.61 ± 1.03	88.66 ± 1.75	84.82 ± 5.73	88.66 ± 1.86	93.57 ± 1.13
XuZhou	ACC	74.14 ± 1.15	77.92 ± 1.08	75.58 ± 0.56	75.55 ± 1.00	76.70 ± 0.77	77.91 ± 0.74	78.23 ± 1.12	80.74 ± 0.89
	NMI	68.48 ± 1.37	72.94 ± 1.34	70.21 ± 0.64	70.81 ± 1.27	72.08 ± 0.90	73.13 ± 0.86	73.34 ± 1.37	76.29 ± 1.04
	ARI	73.03 ± 1.34	74.85 ± 0.67	75.94 ± 0.45	73.12 ± 1.36	74.44 ± 1.04	76.02 ± 0.80	75.24 ± 0.48	77.93 ± 1.07
	Kappa	67.86 ± 1.09	69.53 ± 0.38	69.34 ± 1.12	69.78 ± 2.18	70.11 ± 2.21	71.83 ± 2.13	69.69 ± 0.38	74.92 ± 2.33

2.4.6 Parameter Analysis

(1) *Impact of Hyper-parameters w and M*: The hyperparameter w determines the spatial extent around anchor points, while M regulates the quantity of superpixels. Anchors are positioned at the centroid of each superpixel, ensuring a one-to-one correspondence between superpixels and anchors. Key insights from Fig. 2.10 include: (i) Model performance on the Pavia and XuZhou datasets is highly sensitive to the number of superpixels, likely due to their lower homogeneity, necessitating finer segmentation for optimal results, (ii) Incorporating neighborhood spatial features significantly enhances model accuracy. With spectral data alone ($w = 1$), performance is suboptimal across all datasets. Expanding the neighborhood captures richer spatial context, improving the model's representation. However, excessively large w values degrade accuracy, possibly because broader neighborhoods dilute discriminative information by incorporating irrelevant noise from adjacent samples.

(2) *Impact of Hyper-parameter σ*: Eq. (2.19) incorporates the hyperparameters σ_1 and σ_2 to weight the clustering consistency loss and contrastive learning loss, respectively. Figure 2.11 illustrates the accuracy trends of SSGCC across four datasets as σ varies from 0.1 to 10,000. The results demonstrate that SSGCC maintains stable performance over a broad range of σ_1 and σ_2 values, suggesting robustness to these parameters on certain datasets. Notably, the Pavia University dataset exhibits significant accuracy gains when $\sigma_2 \geq 100$. This improvement can be attributed to the dataset's inherent heterogeneity and the presence of challenging samples. The proposed hard sample mining strategy effectively leverages these conditions, substantially boosting clustering efficacy.

(3) *Impact of Hyper-parameter β*: The hyper-parameter β governs the weighting ratio of sample pairs in our model. Figure 2.12 presents the performance metrics of SSGCC across four datasets as β increases from 1 to 4 in unit increments. Our analysis reveals two critical observations: (i) With insufficient β values, the model assigns excessive weight to simple samples, resulting in suboptimal performance. (ii) Conversely, excessively large β values effectively eliminate the contribution of simple samples, similarly degrading model accuracy. This demonstrates that completely disregarding simple samples adversely affects overall performance. Based on these findings, we empirically determined the optimal β values for each dataset: 2 (Pavia and XuZhou) and 3 (remaining two datasets).

(4) *Impact of Hyper-parameter k*: The hyper-parameter k is the number of neighbors. Figure 2.13 shows the ACC of SSGCC on four datasets when k varies from 15 to 60 with a step size of 5. The findings indicate that when k is too small, the model misses crucial neighbor information, leading to an insufficient capacity to capture remote spatial information, which negatively impacts accuracy. Conversely, when k is too large, it tends to introduce noise, which also degrades the model's performance. Finally, we set k to 45, 50, 50, and 45 on the four datasets.

Fig. 2.10 The sensitivity analysis of two hyper-parameters M and w

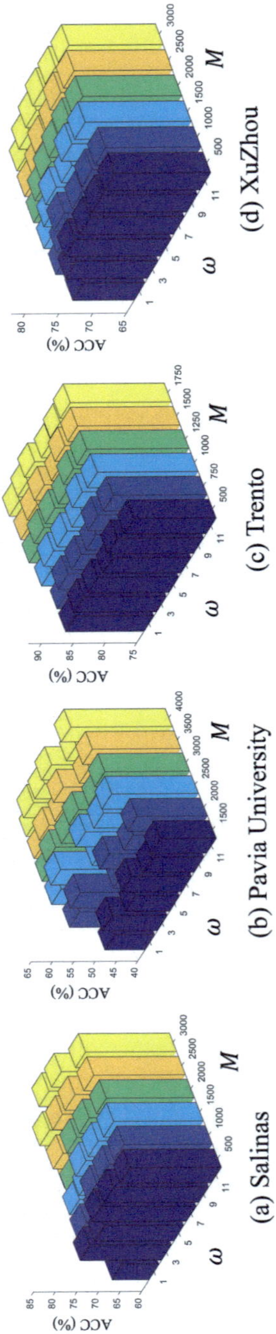

Fig. 2.11 The sensitivity analysis of two hyper-parameters σ_1 and σ_2

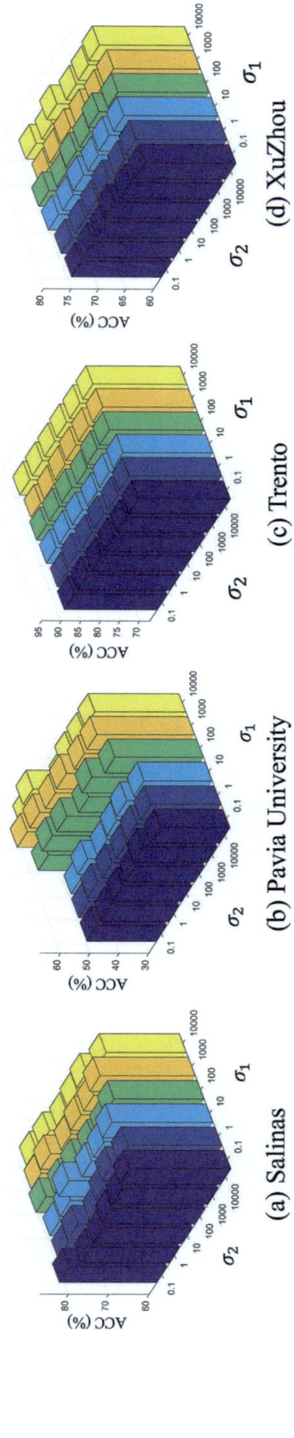

Fig. 2.12 The sensitivity analysis of hyper-parameters β

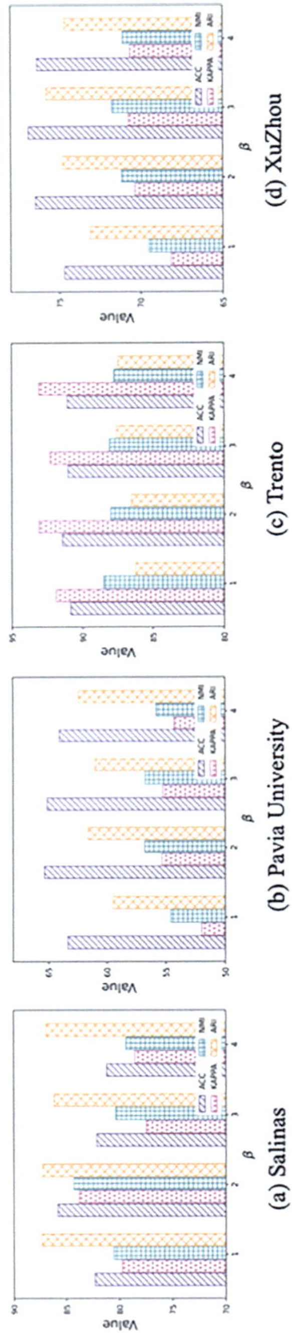

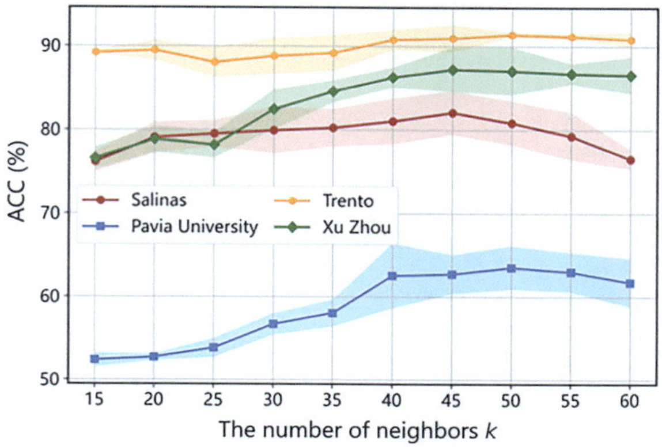

Fig. 2.13 The sensitivity analysis of hyper-parameter *k*

2.5 Conclusion

This chapter introduces SSGCC, a novel deep learning framework for hyperspectral image clustering. The proposed method employs two key components: (i) superpixel-based anchor point selection combined with graph autoencoder (GAE) feature extraction to obtain joint spatial-spectral representations, and (ii) a cluster-aware consistency learning mechanism that enhances node semantics by aligning similarity structures from both spatial and spectral domains. To further improve discrimination capability, we develop an adaptive contrastive learning strategy incorporating hard sample mining. This approach dynamically adjusts sample weights during training, focusing model attention on more challenging instances rather than employing uniform treatment. Experimental evaluations demonstrate SSGCC's superior clustering performance across four benchmark HSI datasets compared to existing methods. Looking ahead, we plan to extend this work by investigating multi-modal remote sensing image clustering. This future direction will focus on leveraging complementary information across different data modalities to achieve more robust clustering performance.

References

1. Ma L, Liu Y, Zhang X, Ye Y, Yin G, Johnson BA (2019) Deep learning in remote sensing applications: a meta-analysis and review. ISPRS J Photogramm Remote Sens 152:166–177
2. Chen Y, Yuan Q, Tang Y, Xiao Y, He J, Liu Z (2024) Sense: Hyperspectral video object tracker via fusing material and motion cues. Inf Fusion 109:102395
3. Liu J, Guan R, Li Z, Zhang J, Hu Y, Wang X (2023) Adaptive multi-feature fusion graph convolutional network for hyperspectral image classification. Remote Sens 15(23):5483
4. Wang C, Guo Y, Fu J (2024) Dual-stream discriminative attention network for cross-scene hyperspectral image classification. IEEE Trans Geosci Remote Sens 62:1–12

5. Chen Z, Lu Z, Gao H, Zhang Y, Zhao J, Hong D, Zhang B (2022) Global to local: A hierarchical detection algorithm for hyperspectral image target detection. IEEE Trans Geosci Remote Sens 60:1–15
6. Zhang X, Wang Z, Li J, Hua Z (2024) Mvafg: multiview fusion and advanced feature guidance change detection network for remote sensing images. IEEE J Select Top Appl Earth Observ Rem Sens 17:11050–11068
7. Yao D, Zhi-li Z, Xiao-feng Z, Wei C, Fang H, Yao-ming C, Cai W-W (2023) Deep hybrid: multi-graph neural network collaboration for hyperspectral image classification. Defence Technol 23:164–176
8. Guan R, Li Z, Li T, Li X, Yang J, Chen W (2022) Classification of heterogeneous mining areas based on rescapsnet and gaofen-5 imagery. Remote Sens 14(13):3216
9. Chen Y, Yuan Q, Tang Y, Xiao Y, He J, Zhang L (2024) Spirit: Spectral awareness interaction network with dynamic template for hyperspectral object tracking. IEEE Trans Geosci Remote Sens 62:1–16
10. Huang R, Xu Y, Hong D, Yao W, Ghamisi P, Stilla U (2020) Deep point embedding for urban classification using als point clouds: A new perspective from local to global. ISPRS J Photogramm Remote Sens 163:62–81
11. Chen Y, Yuan Q, Tang Y, Xiao Y, He J, Han T, Liu Z, Zhang L (2024) Ssttrack: a unified hyperspectral video tracking framework via modeling spectral-spatial-temporal conditions. Inf Fusion 102658
12. Zhai H, Zhang H, Li P, Zhang L (2021) Hyperspectral image clustering: Current achievements and future lines. IEEE Geosci Remote Sens Mag 9(4):35–67
13. Qin Y, Bruzzone L, Li B (2020) Learning discriminative embedding for hyperspectral image clustering based on set-to-set and sample-to-sample distances. IEEE Trans Geosci Remote Sens 58(1):473–485
14. Zhao Y, Li X (2023) Deep spectral clustering with regularized linear embedding for hyperspectral image clustering. IEEE Trans Geosci Remote Sens 61:1–11
15. Shahi KR, Ghamisi P, Rasti B, Gloaguen R, Scheunders P (2022) Ms2a-net: multiscale spectral–spatial association network for hyperspectral image clustering. IEEE J Select Top Appl Earth Observ Rem Sens 15:6518–6530
16. Hao Z, Lu Z, Li G, Nie F, Wang R, Li X (2024) Ensemble clustering with attentional representation. IEEE Trans Knowl Data Eng 36(2):581–593
17. Tu W, Zhou S, Liu X, Guo X, Cai Z, Zhu E, Cheng J (2021) Deep fusion clustering network. Proc AAAI Conf Artif Intell 35(11):9978–9987
18. Luo F, Liu Y, Gong X, Nan Z, Guo T (2024) EMVCC: enhanced multi-view contrastive clustering for hyperspectral images. In: ACM multimedia
19. Liu S, Wang H (2022) Graph convolutional optimal transport for hyperspectral image spectral clustering. IEEE Trans Geosci Remote Sens 60:1–13
20. Wei L, Chen Z, Yin J, Zhu C, Zhou R, Liu J (2023) Adaptive graph convolutional subspace clustering. In: Proceedings of the IEEE/CVF conference on computer vision and pattern recognition, pp 6262–6271
21. Matsushima S, Brbic M (2019) Selective sampling-based scalable sparse subspace clustering. In: Advances in neural information processing systems, vol 32
22. Chen J, Liu S, Zhang Z, Wang H (2023) Diffusion subspace clustering for hyperspectral images. IEEE J Select Top Appl Earth Observ Rem Sens
23. Cai Y, Zeng M, Cai Z, Liu X, Zhang Z (2021) Graph regularized residual subspace clustering network for hyperspectral image clustering. Inf Sci 578:85–101
24. Ding Y, Zhang Z, Zhao X, Cai Y, Li S, Deng B, Cai W (2022) Self-supervised locality preserving low-pass graph convolutional embedding for large-scale hyperspectral image clustering. IEEE Trans Geosci Remote Sens 60:1–16
25. Han T, Niu S, Gao X, Yu W, Cui N, Dong J (2022) Deep low-rank graph convolutional subspace clustering for hyperspectral image. IEEE Trans Geosci Remote Sens 60:1–13
26. Zhang Y, Wang Y, Chen X, Jiang X, Zhou Y (2022) Spectral–spatial feature extraction with dual graph autoencoder for hyperspectral image clustering. IEEE Trans Circuits Syst Video Technol 32(12):8500–8511

27. Peng B, Yao Y, Lei J, Fang L, Huang Q (2023) Graph-based structural deep spectral-spatial clustering for hyperspectral image. IEEE Trans Instrum Meas 72:1–12
28. Zhang Z, Ding Y, Zhao X, Siye L, Yang N, Cai Y, Zhan Y (2023) Multireceptive field: An adaptive path aggregation graph neural framework for hyperspectral image classification. Expert Syst Appl 217:119508
29. Ding Y, Zhang Z, Zhao X, Hong D, Cai W, Yang N, Wang B (2023) Multi-scale receptive fields: graph attention neural network for hyperspectral image classification. Expert Syst Appl 223:119858
30. Cai Y, Zhang Z, Liu X, Ding Y, Li F, Tan J (2024) Learning unified anchor graph for joint clustering of hyperspectral and lidar data. IEEE Trans Neural Netw Learn Syst 1–14
31. Tu W, Zhou S, Liu X, Liu Y, Cai Z, Zhu E, Zhang C, Cheng J (2022) Initializing then refining: a simple graph attribute imputation network. In Proceedings of the twenty-fourth international joint conference on artificial intelligence (IJCAI), pp 3494–3500
32. Tu W, Liao Q, Zhou S, Peng X, Ma C, Liu Z, Liu X, Cai Z (2023) Rare: robust masked graph autoencoder. In: IEEE transactions on knowledge and data engineering (IEEE TKDE), pp 1–14
33. Cai Y, Zhang Z, Liu Y, Ghamisi P, Li K, Liu X, Cai Z (2021) Large-scale hyperspectral image clustering using contrastive learning. arXiv preprint arXiv:2111.07945
34. Hu X, Li T, Zhou T, Peng Y (2021) Deep spatial-spectral subspace clustering for hyperspectral images based on contrastive learning. Remote Sens 13(21):4418
35. Cai Y, Zhang Z, Ghamisi P, Ding Y, Liu X, Cai Z, Gloaguen R (2022) Superpixel contracted neighborhood contrastive subspace clustering network for hyperspectral images. IEEE Trans Geosci Remote Sens 60:1–13
36. Guan R, Li Z, Li X, Tang C (2024) Pixel-superpixel contrastive learning and pseudo-label correction for hyperspectral image clustering. In: ICASSP 2024–2024 IEEE international conference on acoustics, speech and signal processing (ICASSP). IEEE, pp 6795–6799
37. Huang S, Zeng H, Chen H, Zhang H (2024) Spatial and cluster structural prior guided subspace clustering for hyperspectral image. IEEE Trans Geosci Remote Sens
38. Guan R, Li Z, Tu W, Wang J, Liu Y, Li X, Tang C, Feng R (2024) Contrastive multiview subspace clustering of hyperspectral images based on graph convolutional networks. IEEE Trans Geosci Remote Sens 62:1–14
39. Tu W, Zhou S, Liu X, Ge C, Cai Z, Liu Y (2023) Hierarchically contrastive hard sample mining for graph self-supervised pretraining. IEEE Trans Neural Netw Learn Syst 1–14
40. Bezdek JC (2013) Pattern recognition with fuzzy objective function algorithms. Springer Science & Business Media
41. Kanungo T, Mount DM, Netanyahu NS, Piatko CD, Silverman R, Wu AY (2002) An efficient k-means clustering algorithm: analysis and implementation. IEEE Trans Pattern Anal Mach Intell 24(7):881–892
42. Rafiezadeh Shahi K, Khodadadzadeh M, Tusa L, Ghamisi P, Tolosana-Delgado R, Gloaguen R (2020) Hierarchical sparse subspace clustering (HESSC): an automatic approach for hyperspectral image analysis. Remote Sens 12(15):2421
43. Huang K, Li X, Pi Y, Cheng H, Xu G (2023) Graph-constrained residual self-expressive subspace clustering network for hyperspectral images. IEEE J Select Top Appl Earth Observ Rem Sens 17:941–955
44. Luo F, Liu Y, Duan Y, Guo T, Zhang L, Du B (2024) Sdst: Self-supervised double-structure transformer for hyperspectral images clustering. IEEE Trans Geosci Remote Sens
45. Cui K, Li R, Polk SL, Lin Y, Zhang H, Murphy JM, Plemmons RJ, Chan RH (2024) Superpixel-based and spatially regularized diffusion learning for unsupervised hyperspectral image clustering. IEEE Trans Geosci Remote Sens 62:1–18
46. Zhao H, Zhou F, Bruzzone L, Guan R, Yang C (2022) Superpixel-level global and local similarity graph-based clustering for large hyperspectral images. IEEE Trans Geosci Remote Sens 60:1–16
47. Huang N, Xiao L, Liu Q, Chanussot J (2023) S2dmsc: A self-supervised deep multilevel subspace clustering approach for large hyperspectral images. IEEE Trans Geosci Remote Sens 61:1–17

48. Ding Y, Zhang Z, Zhao X, Cai W, Yang N, Hu H, Huang X, Cao Y, Cai W (2022) Unsupervised self-correlated learning smoothy enhanced locality preserving graph convolution embedding clustering for hyperspectral images. IEEE Trans Geosci Remote Sens 60:1–16
49. Zhang Z, Liu Y, Xiao M, Wang K, Huang Y, Bian J, Yang R, Li F (2024) Graph contrastive learning as a versatile foundation for advanced scrna-seq data analysis, pp 2024–04
50. Liu Y, Zhang Z, Qin S, Salim FD, Yepes AJ (2023) Contrastive learning-based imputation-prediction networks for in-hospital mortality risk modeling using EHRS. In: Joint European conference on machine learning and knowledge discovery in databases, pp 428–443
51. Liu Y, Yang X, Zhou S, Liu X, Wang S, Liang K, Tu W, Li L (2023) Simple contrastive graph clustering. IEEE Trans Neural Netw Learn Syst 1–12
52. Tu W, Guan R, Zhou S, Ma C, Peng X, Cai Z, Liu Z, Cheng J, Liu X (2024) Attribute-missing graph clustering network. In: Proceedings of the AAAI conference on artificial intelligence, vol 38, no 14, pp 15392–15401
53. Hu D, Dong Z, Liang K, Yu H, Wang S, Liu X (2024) High-order topology for deep single-cell multi-view fuzzy clustering. IEEE Trans Fuzzy Syst
54. Hu D, Liang K, Dong Z, Wang J, Zhao Y, He K (2024) Effective multi-modal clustering method via skip aggregation network for parallel SCRNA-SEQ and SCATAC-SEQ data. Brief Bioinf 25(2):102
55. Oord Avd, Li Y, Vinyals O (2018) Representation learning with contrastive predictive coding. arXiv preprint arXiv:1807.03748
56. Guan R, Li Z, Song C, Yu G, Li X, Feng R (2024) S2rc-gcn: a spatial-spectral reliable contrastive graph convolutional network for complex land cover classification using hyperspectral images. arXiv preprint arXiv:2404.00964
57. Wang J, Guan R, Gao K, Li Z, Li H, Li X, Tang C (2024) Multi-level graph subspace contrastive learning for hyperspectral image clustering. arXiv preprint arXiv:2404.05211
58. Li J, Guan R, Han Y, Hu Y, Li Z, Wu Y, Xu Z, Li X (2024) Superpixel-based dual-neighborhood contrastive graph autoencoder for deep subspace clustering of hyperspectral image. In: International conference on intelligent computing. Springer, pp 181–192
59. Cai Y, Zhang Z, Ghamisi P, Rasti B, Liu X, Cai Z (2023) Transformer-based contrastive prototypical clustering for multimodal remote sensing data. Inf Sci 649:119655
60. Qi J, Jia Y, Liu H, Hou J (2024) Superpixel graph contrastive clustering with semantic-invariant augmentations for hyperspectral images. arXiv preprint arXiv:2403.01799
61. Kalantidis Y, Sariyildiz MB, Pion N, Weinzaepfel P, Larlus D (2020) Hard negative mixing for contrastive learning. Adv Neural Inf Proces Syst 33:21798–21809
62. Liu Y, Yang X, Zhou S, Liu X, Wang Z, Liang K, Tu W, Li L, Duan J, Chen C (2023) Hard sample aware network for contrastive deep graph clustering. Proc AAAI Conf Artif Intell 37(7):8914–8922
63. Liang K, Liu Y, Zhou S, Tu W, Wen Y, Yang X, Dong X, Liu X (2023) Knowledge graph contrastive learning based on relation-symmetrical structure. IEEE Trans Knowl Data Eng 36(1):226–238
64. Hao Z, Xin H, Wei L, Tang L, Wang R, Nie F (2024) Towards expansive and adaptive hard negative mining: graph contrastive learning via subspace preserving. Proc ACM Web Conf 2024:322–333
65. Zhang C, Zhang K, Pham TX, Niu A, Qiao Z, Yoo CD, Kweon IS (2022) Dual temperature helps contrastive learning without many negative samples: towards understanding and simplifying moco. In: Proceedings of the IEEE/CVF conference on computer vision and pattern recognition (CVPR), pp 14441–14450
66. Xia J, Wu L, Wang G, Chen J, Li SZ (2022) Progcl: Rethinking hard negative mining in graph contrastive learning. In: International conference on machine learning, pp 24332–24346
67. Rodarmel C, Shan J (2002) Principal component analysis for hyperspectral image classification. Surv Land Inf Sci 62(2):115–122
68. Achanta R, Shaji A, Smith K, Lucchi A, Fua P, Susstrunk S (2012) SLIC superpixels compared to state-of-the-art superpixel methods. IEEE Trans Pattern Anal Mach Intell 34(11):2274–2282

69. Elhamifar E, Vidal R (2013) Sparse subspace clustering: algorithm, theory, and applications. IEEE Trans Pattern Anal Mach Intell 35(11):2765–2781
70. Baldi P (2012) Autoencoders, unsupervised learning, and deep architectures. In: Proceedings of ICML workshop on unsupervised and transfer learning. In: JMLR workshop and conference proceedings, pp 37–49
71. Xie J, Girshick R, Farhadi A (2016) Unsupervised deep embedding for clustering analysis. In: International conference on machine learning. PMLR 478–487
72. Guo X, Gao L, Liu X, Yin J (2017) Improved deep embedded clustering with local structure preservation. IJCAI 17:1753–1759
73. Quan H, Li X, Hu D, Nan T, Cui X (2024) Dual-channel prototype network for few-shot pathology image classification. IEEE J Biomed Health Inf
74. Meng L, Liang K, Xiao B, Zhou S, Liu Y, Liu M, Yang X, Liu X, Li J (2024) SARF: aliasing relation–assisted self-supervised learning for few-shot relation reasoning. IEEE Trans Neural Netw Learn Syst 1–11
75. Liu M, Liu Y, Liang K, Tu W, Wang S, Zhou S, Liu X (2024) Deep temporal graph clustering. In: The 12th international conference on learning representations
76. Liu M, Liang K, Zhao Y, Tu W, Zhou S, Gan X, Liu X, Kunlun H (2024) Self-supervised temporal graph learning with temporal and structural intensity alignment. IEEE Trans Neural Netw Learn Syst
77. Liang K, Meng L, Liu M, Liu Y, Tu W, Wang S, Zhou S, Liu X, Sun F, He K (2024) A survey of knowledge graph reasoning on graph types: Static, dynamic, and multi-modal. IEEE Trans Pattern Anal Mach Intell 1–20
78. Li R, Hu Y, Li L, Guan R, Yang R, Zhan J, Cai W, Wang Y, Xu H, Li L (2024) SMWE-GFPNNET: a high-precision and robust method for forest fire smoke detection. Knowl-Based Syst 289:111528
79. Hu T, Yan Q, Qi Y, Zhang Y (2024) Generating content for HDR deghosting from frequency view. In: Proceedings of the IEEE/CVF conference on computer vision and pattern recognition, pp 25732–25741
80. Yan Q, Hu T, Sun Y, Tang H, Zhu Y, Dong W, Van Gool L, Zhang Y (2023) Towards high-quality HDR deghosting with conditional diffusion models. IEEE Trans Circuit Syst Video Technol 34:4011–4026

Chapter 3
Multi-view Subspace Graph Convolutional Clustering for Hyperspectral Images

3.1 Introduction

Recent advances in spectral imaging have established hyperspectral imagery (HSI) as a powerful analytical tool, driving innovation across multiple scientific and operational domains. These high-resolution spectral datasets have demonstrated particular value in environmental monitoring [1], security applications [2], and geological exploration [3, 4]. Compared to traditional RGB imaging systems, HSI captures significantly richer spectral signatures while maintaining superior spatial resolution, enabling more accurate surface characterization [5, 6]. These distinctive capabilities have spurred the creation of numerous specialized processing methods tailored for hyperspectral data analysis [7].

Recent decades have witnessed substantial progress in supervised hyperspectral image (HSI) classification, ranging from conventional machine learning approaches like support vector machines [10] to advanced deep learning architectures, including convolutional neural networks (CNNs) and transformer-based models [11]. While effective, these supervised methods depend heavily on manually annotated training data, which demands significant human effort and specialized knowledge [12]. To overcome the challenges of limited labeled data and reduce annotation burdens, unsupervised learning techniques—particularly clustering—have emerged as a promising alternative [13, 14]. Clustering facilitates automated HSI analysis by grouping pixels with similar spectral-spatial characteristics. Nevertheless, the high spectral variability and complex spatial patterns inherent in HSI data present considerable challenges for clustering algorithms [15].

HSI clustering involves grouping pixels into distinct categories by maximizing intra-class similarity while minimizing inter-class variance [16]. Existing clustering algorithms can be broadly categorized into: (i) Centroid-based methods, such as k-means [17] and fuzzy c-means [18], which iteratively optimize cluster centers; (ii) Density-based approaches, including mean shift [19] and ensemble density analysis

Y. Ding et al., *Graph Neural Network for Hyperspectral Image Clustering*, Intelligent Perception and Information Processing, https://doi.org/10.1007/978-981-96-7710-8_3

[20], which utilize spatial feature distribution; and (iii) Subspace clustering techniques [21–24], which exploit the underlying data structure for improved performance. While effective, traditional methods exhibit limitations in robustness, as they are sensitive to initialization parameters, noise interference, and predefined similarity metrics. Subspace clustering has emerged as a particularly promising direction, demonstrating superior capability in capturing the intrinsic characteristics of HSI data.

Subspace clustering algorithms effectively integrate traditional feature selection techniques with clustering approaches to process feature subsets or weights corresponding to each data cluster during the partitioning of samples [25]. Notable examples include sparse subspace clustering (SSC) [26] and low-rank subspace clustering [27], which rely on identifying the sparse representation matrix of the original data, constructing a similarity graph on the corresponding matrix, and employing spectral clustering to derive clustering outcomes. Recent advances have focused on better leveraging the spatial-spectral information inherent in HSI data cubes. Zhang et al. [26] developed an SSC-based approach that significantly improves clustering accuracy. Further enhancements include the l_2-SSC algorithm [28], which incorporates neighborhood information through l_2-norm regularization, and Huang's semi-supervised method [29] that employs joint constraints to better utilize local spatial information. These innovations have collectively advanced subspace clustering performance for HSI applications.

Although traditional subspace clustering methods have achieved reasonable performance, their effectiveness in complex HSI scenarios remains limited by inherent constraints. In contrast, deep clustering approaches have demonstrated superior capability in learning robust and discriminative feature representations [16, 30–32]. First, autoencoder-based architectures have shown promise, exemplified by Lei et al. [33], who employed stacked autoencoders for self-expression learning to enhance feature extraction. Building on this foundation, self-supervised methods have further advanced the field, with Li et al. [34] integrating adaptive initialization to achieve state-of-the-art clustering performance. Further progress has been made through the incorporation of graph-based techniques. Cai et al. [35] developed the GR-RSCNet framework, which combines deep residual learning with graph regularization to improve nonlinear affinity modeling. The success of graph convolutional networks has been particularly noteworthy, as they naturally capture neighborhood relationships in HSI data. This is illustrated by Cai et al. [36] through their graph convolutional subspace clustering (GCSC) method, which effectively integrates structural and attribute information. More recently, researchers have explored higher-order relationships using hypergraph convolution, with Zhang et al. [37, 38] demonstrating its effectiveness in modeling complex dependencies within HSI data. Collectively, these deep learning approaches have significantly advanced subspace clustering by simultaneously addressing three critical aspects: robust feature extraction, sophisticated relationship modeling, and nonlinear representation learning. The integration of these capabilities has led to substantial improvements in clustering accuracy and robustness, particularly for challenging HSI applications.

Despite advancements in clustering performance, existing algorithms still face two critical limitations. First, their direct application to hyperspectral images (HSIs) often results in noisy cluster maps, primarily due to three factors: (1) limited discriminative information in the spectral domain, (2) the complexity of ground objects, and (3) intra-class spectral heterogeneity [39]. Second, most methods operate on a single view, despite extensive evidence demonstrating that multi-view complementary information can significantly improve clustering accuracy [40–42]. Recent efforts to address these challenges have explored multi-view clustering frameworks. For instance, Tian et al. [43] proposed a multi-view approach, though it remained sensitive to noise. Chen et al. [44] applied multi-view subspace clustering to polarized HSI data, employing pre-clustering for sparse representation across views. Huang et al. [45] enhanced clustering performance by combining local and non-local spatial information to identify a shared intrinsic cluster structure. Similarly, Lu et al. [46] fused spectral and spatial features using multi-view kernels for collaborative subspace clustering, achieving superior results. While these methods demonstrate the potential of multi-view information, they exhibit notable shortcomings. Most critically, they fail to leverage cross-view guidance during feature learning and neglect to weight the contributions of distinct views. This oversight can lead to the loss of critical information, as the relative importance of spectral, spatial, or other view-specific features remains unoptimized.

To overcome these limitations, this study proposes an innovative multi-view subspace clustering framework designed for hyperspectral images, integrating both textural and spectral-spatial features. The approach employs a graph convolutional network alongside contrastive learning strategies [47, 48] to capture local neighborhood data while enhancing cross-view consistency in feature representation. An attention-based adaptive fusion mechanism further refines the affinity matrices, yielding a more distinctive clustering output. The key contributions of this work include:

1. This study introduces CMSCGC, an innovative deep multi-view subspace clustering framework specifically designed for hyperspectral image analysis. The proposed method simultaneously processes both textural and spectral-spatial features to enhance clustering performance.
2. By incorporating contrastive learning, CMSCGC enhances cross-view representation consistency, improving the model's ability to derive discriminative and stable feature embeddings.
3. The proposed framework employs an attention-based fusion mechanism to dynamically integrate affinity matrices, generating a more refined and discriminative representation for clustering.
4. Extensive experiments conducted on four benchmark datasets confirm that the proposed approach achieves superior performance compared to existing state-of-the-art methods.
5. Sect. 3.2 surveys foundational concepts in multi-view subspace clustering, hyperspectral image analysis, and contrastive learning frameworks. The proposed CMSCGC methodology is comprehensively detailed in Sect. 3.3. Experimental

results and comparative analyses are presented in Sect. 3.4, with final conclusions and implications discussed in Sect. 3.5.

3.2 Related Work

This section begins by examining core principles and architectures in multi-view subspace clustering. Subsequently, we discuss key advancements in hyperspectral image clustering techniques and contrastive learning paradigms, highlighting their evolving methodologies and applications.

3.2.1 Multi-view Subspace Clustering

Current multi-view clustering techniques [48–51] have demonstrated significant effectiveness in diverse application domains. These methods show particular promise for remote sensing image analysis [38], where the integration of complementary multi-view data can substantially enhance clustering performance. Given multi-view data $\{X^p\}_{p=1}^{P}$, where $X^p \in R^{d^p \times n}$ denotes the p-th view data with an upper dimension of d^p and n is the number of samples, subspace clustering postulates that every point can be expressed by a linear combination of other points within the same subspace. Based on this assumption, data X^p for each view were employed as a dictionary to construct the subspace representation model as follows:

$$X^p = X^p C^p + E^p \tag{3.1}$$

where $C^p \in R^{n \times n}$ and E^p represent the self-expression matrix for each view and representation error. Multi-view subspace clustering methods are typically described as follows:

$$\begin{aligned} &\min_{C^p} \left\| X^p - X^p C^p \right\|_F^2 + \lambda f\left(C^p\right) \\ &\text{s.t. } C^p \geq 0,\ C^{p^T} 1 = 1, \end{aligned} \tag{3.2}$$

where $C^{p^T} 1 = 1$ ensures that the sum of each column in C^p is 1, indicating that every sample point can be reconstructed through a linear combination of the other samples. $C^p_{i,j}$ represents the weight of the edge between the i-th and j-th samples. Hence, C^p can be viewed as an n × n undirected graph and $\|\cdot\|_F$ represents applying Frobenius norm to the matrix and $f(\cdot)$ is a regularization function, and λ is a parameter that balances regularization and loss. Different $f(\cdot)$ functions yield self-expression matrices C^p that satisfy various constraints. For instance, sparse constraints have been applied to matrices [26] or low-rank representations of data [27].

Upon obtaining self-expression matrices $\{C^p\}_{p=1}^{P}$ for each view, they are fused to create a unified self-expression matrix $C^p \in R^{n \times n}$. In certain methods, this step is performed concurrently with the learning phase across all the views. Using a consistent C^p as the input for spectral clustering yields the final clustering outcome. The spectral clustering framework initially requires building a similarity matrix, which conventionally involves pairwise sample comparisons. This process leads to quadratic computational complexity, with both time and space requirements scaling as $O(n^2)$ where n represents the number of data points. Then proceed to compute the eigenvectors of the Laplacian matrix, which has a time complexity of $O(n^3)$ for dense matrices. Therefore, the overall time complexity of Eq. (3.2) is $O(n^3)$.

3.2.2 Hyperspectral Image Clustering

The analysis of hyperspectral imagery presents significant challenges due to its inherent high dimensionality, strong band correlations, and non-linear data distributions. Conventional supervised classification approaches demand extensive labeled training samples, which are frequently scarce or costly to acquire. To address this constraint, unsupervised clustering techniques for hyperspectral images (HSIs) have emerged as a prominent research direction. These methods automatically categorize pixels into distinct groups based on spectral similarity, eliminating the need for prior label information. While classical clustering approaches like k-means remain popular due to their computational efficiency and straightforward implementation, they often produce inconsistent and suboptimal results when applied to complex hyperspectral datasets.

Subspace clustering has emerged as one of the most effective approaches for hyperspectral image (HSI) analysis due to its strong robustness. Techniques such as sparse and low-rank subspace clustering [26, 27] are notable examples, though traditional methods often overlook valuable non-spectral data. To address this limitation, researchers have increasingly focused on incorporating spatial features. For example, Zhang et al. [52] developed a robust manifold matrix factorization (RMMF) method by integrating spatial-spectral correlations within a non-negative matrix factorization framework, achieving significant improvements. Similarly, Cai et al. [36] enhanced subspace clustering by applying graph convolutional networks (GCNs), enabling better fusion of clustering and feature extraction. Further advancements were made by Liu et al. [53], who optimized graph representation learning through an optimal transport strategy, boosting the efficacy of graph-based subspace clustering.

3.2.3 Contrastive Learning

Contrastive learning is a self-supervised approach that acquires meaningful feature representations by distinguishing between positive and negative data instances. The core principle involves training a model to assess the relationships between sample pairs by projecting them into a shared latent space, where their proximity is quantified using distance metrics [54]. This framework encourages the model to minimize divergence among similar inputs while maximizing separation for dissimilar ones.

Contrastive learning has found extensive use across diverse domains, particularly in computer vision applications [55]. A notable example is SimCLR [56], a foundational framework that enhances feature extraction by enforcing similarity between differently augmented versions of the same input, highlighting the crucial role of data transformations in this paradigm. Another significant contribution is MoCo [57], which formulates contrastive learning as a dynamic dictionary retrieval task, maintaining computational efficiency while reducing memory overhead. Further advancing this field, Gansbeke et al. [55] introduced the SCAN method, where initial clusters derived from pretrained features guide subsequent learning by leveraging nearest-neighbor relationships. In contrast, BYOL [58] achieves representation learning solely through positive pair alignment, eliminating the need for negative samples. Similarly, Simsiam [59] prevents degenerate solutions through gradient cutoff mechanisms. Recent innovations include Barlow Twins [60], which optimizes feature invariance by aligning cross-correlation matrices with identity matrices. Additionally, graph-based contrastive approaches [61, 62] have emerged, significantly advancing unsupervised representation learning for structured data. These developments collectively demonstrate the versatility and effectiveness of contrastive techniques across different data modalities.

Recent advances have extended contrastive learning techniques to remote sensing applications [63]. Several innovative approaches demonstrate this trend: Hou et al. [64] developed an unsupervised framework to extract discriminative features from hyperspectral imagery for improved classification performance. Wang et al. [65] implemented a semi-supervised contrastive clustering approach, utilizing high-confidence pseudo-labels for change detection in satellite imagery. For semantic segmentation tasks, Li et al. [66] introduced a dual-scale contrastive method that captures both global and local features. In a multimodal approach, Wang et al. [67] effectively combined hyperspectral and LiDAR data through contrastive learning for enhanced classification accuracy. Notably, current literature reveals a research gap in applying multi-view contrastive learning to hyperspectral image clustering. Our proposed framework addresses this limitation by enforcing feature consistency across different views while maximizing similarity among samples from identical land-cover categories. This strategy significantly improves feature discrimination and clustering robustness, as quantitatively validated in Sect. 3.4.

3.3 Proposed Method

As illustrated in Fig. 3.1, our proposed system comprises four key modules: multi-view graph generation, graph convolutional self-expression, contrastive feature learning, and attention-based fusion. The subsequent sections first detail the multi-view graph formulation process, then systematically present the remaining components. For reference, all mathematical notations are comprehensively defined in Table 3.1.

3.3.1 *Multi-view Graph Construction*

This component aims to generate multi-view graphs by capturing both textural characteristics and spatial-spectral relationships. Prior to graph construction, we first address the inherent challenge of hyperspectral data redundancy through dimensionality reduction. Principal component analysis (PCA) [68] was applied to compress the high-dimensional bands into a lower-dimensional space. For spatial-spectral feature extraction, we implemented a sliding window approach that processes each pixel along with its local neighborhood. This generates representative patches where each patch corresponds to its central pixel, maintaining a one-to-one correspondence between patches and image pixels [36, 69]. In parallel, we utilized the extended morphological profiles (EMP) technique [40] to transform the spectral data while preserving crucial textural information through successive erosion operations. This dual-path processing enables comprehensive feature representation for subsequent graph construction. Therefore, we can obtain multi-view features $\{X^p\}_{p=1}^P \in R^{d^p \times n}$,

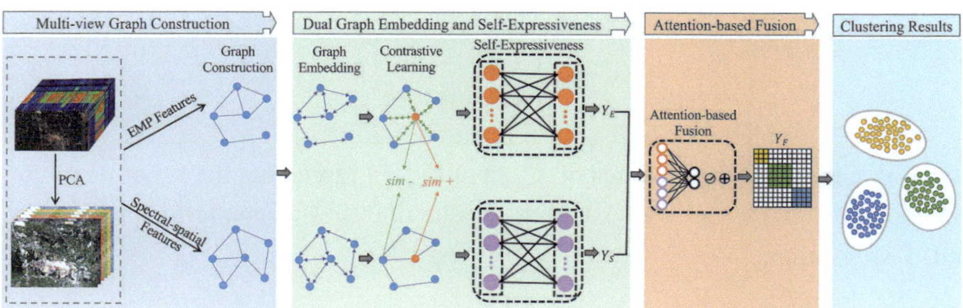

Fig. 3.1 The CMSCGC framework implements a multi-stage processing pipeline for hyperspectral image analysis. The initial phase involves generating multiple graph representations from the original hyperspectral data. These graph structures subsequently undergo feature extraction through a dual-component system combining graph convolutional networks with contrastive learning mechanisms. The derived features are then intelligently aggregated using an attention-based fusion approach to produce a stable affinity matrix. The final stage employs spectral clustering techniques on this optimized matrix to generate the ultimate segmentation results

Table 3.1 Summary of notations

Notation	Description
n	The number of data points
p	The number of views
ω	The input size of the model
k	Number of neighbors selected for each node
d^p	The dimension of X^p
$\hat{d}^p$	The dimension of Z^p
$X^p \in R^{d^p \times n}$	The data matrix on the p-th view
$Z^p \in R^{\hat{d}^p \times n}$	The feature matrix on the p-th view
$C^p \in R^{n \times n}$	The self-expression matrix learned on the p-th view
$A^p \in R^{n \times n}$	The adjacency matrices on the p-th view
$Y^p \in R^{n \times n}$	The affinity matrices on the p-th view

where $x^p \in R^{\omega \times w \times d^p}$, w and p are the patch size and the dimension of each view, respectively.

Because the GCN can only operate directly on graph-structured data, it is necessary to convert the processed data into a topological graph structure. Multi-view graphs can be defined as $G^p = (V^p, E^p, X^p)$ where V^p and E^p are the corresponding node and edge sets, and the edges are denoted by the adjacency matrix A^p. Here, the data in each view are considered nodes of the graph, and the topology is constructed using their K-nearest neighbors. In each view, the adjacency matrices A^p are constructed by measuring the Euclidean distance between the centroids of different patches, which describes the global similarity of the data points. The elements in adjacency matrices A^p can be defined as:

$$A_{i,j}^p = \begin{cases} 1, x_j^p \in N_k\left(x_i^p\right) \\ 0, \text{otherwise} \end{cases} \tag{3.3}$$

where x_i^p and x_j^p are the columns of $A_{i,j}^p$, and $N_k\left(x_i^p\right)$ represents the set of neighbors that include x_i in the p-th view. $A_{i,j}^p$ has a value of 0 or 1, depending on whether x_i^p and x_j^p are similar.

3.3.2 Graph Convolutional Self-expression Module

Current hyperspectral image clustering approaches have largely neglected the critical aspect of topological relationship learning between objects. While conventional convolutional neural networks (CNNs) demonstrate limited capability in capturing these structural patterns, emerging evidence suggests that explicitly modeling object topology could significantly enhance clustering performance. This gap motivates the development of specialized architectures capable of effectively learning and preserving the spatial and contextual relationships inherent in hyperspectral data.

In contrast to CNNs, GCNs effectively capture interdependencies among nodes by leveraging graph-based convolutions, which integrate both node features and structural relationships within the neighborhood. Mathematically, the formula for the spectral graph convolution at the l-th layer is

$$\begin{aligned} H^p(l+1) &= f\left(H^p(l), \tilde{A}^p; W^{(l)}\right) \\ &= \sigma\left(\tilde{D}^{p^{-\frac{1}{2}}} \tilde{A}^p \tilde{D}^{p^{-\frac{1}{2}}} H^p(l) W^p(l)\right) \end{aligned} \tag{3.4}$$

In this equation, $\tilde{A}^p = A^p + I_N$, where I_N is the identity matrix; $\tilde{D}^p$ and $W^p(l)$ represent the degree matrix of nodes in each view and the weight matrix of the $l+1$-th layer, respectively; σ denotes the activation function; $H(l)$ is for the data representation at layer l, and when l equals 0, $H^p(0)$ represents the input multi-view data.

Drawing on the framework for graph convolutional subspace clustering introduced in [36], we adapt the conventional self-expression approach by incorporating a self-expression coefficient matrix, thereby enhancing the robustness of the extracted information as detailed below:

$$X^p = X^p \overline{A}^p C^p = Z^p C^p \text{s.t. } \operatorname{diag}\left(C^p\right) = 0, \tag{3.5}$$

where C^p is the self-expression coefficient matrix for each view, and $X\overline{A}C$ can be regarded as a special linear graph convolution operation parameterized by C, where $\overline{A}$ represents the normalized adjacency matrix. The final graph self-expression is defined as

$$\min_{C^p} \frac{1}{2}(\lambda \left\| Z^p C^p - X \right\|_F^{p2} + \lambda \left\| C^p \right\|_q) \quad \text{st } \operatorname{diag}\left(C^p\right) = 0, \tag{3.6}$$

where q denotes an appropriate matrix norm, and λ is the balancing coefficient. The purpose of graph convolutional self-expression is to reconstruct the original data using a self-expressive coefficient matrix C. As C includes the global structural information, a clearer dictionary can be obtained, generating a robust affinity matrix. By setting $\|\cdot\|_q$ as the Frobenius norm, the self-expression loss function can be obtained as follows:

$$L_{\mathrm{SE}} = \frac{1}{2}\left(\left\|Z^p C^p - X^p\right\|_F^2 + \lambda\left\|C^p\right\|_F\right)$$
$$\frac{1}{2}tr\left[(Z^p C^p - X^p)^T (Z^p C^p - X^p) + \lambda C^{p^T} C^p\right] \tag{3.7}$$

The obtained multi-view self-expression coefficient matrices C^p can be used to construct affinity matrices Y^p:

$$Y^p = \frac{1}{2}\left(\left|C^p\right| + \left|C^p\right|^T\right). \tag{3.8}$$

3.3.3 Contrastive Learning

A key challenge in multi-view clustering lies in efficiently leveraging data from diverse perspectives. This requires the integration of consistent patterns across different views to enhance clustering performance. Building on the previously discussed GCN, which has already captured rich multi-view representations, we now denote the node features as z to streamline further processing.

Recent advances in contrastive learning have shown remarkable effectiveness for clustering applications, primarily due to its ability to preserve data invariance through similarity distribution constraints. The core principle involves: generating positive and negative sample pairs, minimizing distances between positive pairs, and maximizing separation from negative pairs to enhance feature representations. Considerable research has focused on optimizing sample pair construction, as this critically impacts downstream performance. For our framework, we leverage naturally occurring high-quality positive pairs (corresponding nodes across different views) while employing randomly selected inter-graph nodes as negative samples.

For any node i on the graph, we consider its node representation z_i in one view as the anchor point, and the corresponding node representations in the other views, denoted as z_i', form the positive samples. As mentioned earlier, we want z_i to be as far from the negative samples as possible and closer to the positive samples. The loss function is designed as follows:

$$l\left(z_i, z_i'\right) = -\log \frac{e^{\left(\mathrm{sim}\left(z_i z_i'\right)/\tau\right)}}{\sum_{k=1}^{N} e^{\left(\mathrm{sim}\left(z_i z_k'\right)/\tau\right)} + \sum_{k=1}^{N} e^{\left(\mathrm{sim}\left(z_i z_k\right)/\tau\right)}}, \tag{3.9}$$

where τ represents the temperature parameter and it is fixed to 1 in this chapter, $\mathrm{sim}(\cdot)$ is the cosine similarity function, z_i' represents the negative sample representation in other views, and z_i represents the representation of the negative pair within the same layer. The overall objective for minimizing is the average of Eq. (3.9) for all given positive pairs, which is given by the following expression:

$$l_{\text{con}} = \frac{1}{2n}\sum_{i=1}^{n}\left[l\left(z_i, z_i'\right) + l\left(z_i', z_i\right)\right]. \tag{3.10}$$

3.3.4 Attention Fusion Module

After obtaining affinity matrices Y^p from Eq. (3.8), we must fuse them to construct the final affinity graph and apply spectral clustering to the final affinity matrix. We utilized an attention-based fusion module to learn the importance a^p of each view as follows:

$$a^p = \text{att}\left(Y^p\right), \tag{3.11}$$

where $a^p \in R^{n\times 1}$ are used to measure the importance of each view. Details of the attention module are provided below. In the first step, we concatenate affinity matrices Y^p as $\left[Y_1...Y_p\right]$ and introduce a weight matrix $S \in R^{pn\times n}$ to capture the relationships between the self-expression matrices. And S is initialized with the all-ones initialization to endow the same weight to affinity matrices at the beginning of training and the updated S represents the weights of the linear layer. Next, we apply the tan$h$ function to the product of $\left[Y_1...Y_p\right]$ and W for a transformation. Finally, we use softmax and the l_2 function to normalize the attention values, resulting in the final weight matrix

$$a^p = l_2\left(\text{sofmax}\left(\tanh\left(\left[Y_1...Y_p\right] \times S\right)\right)\right). \tag{3.12}$$

The weight matrix can be obtained to realize the fusion operation, and fused self-expression matrix Y_F is

$$Y_F = f\left(Y_1...Y_p\right) = \sum_{i=1}^{N}(a_i 1) \odot Y_i, \tag{3.13}$$

where $1 \in R^{1\times n}$ is a matrix with all elements being 1, and $\odot$ represents the Hadamard product of the matrix.

Algorithm 1: Learning procedure for CMSCGC

Input: HSI data X, the input size w, the number of neighbors: k, the regularization coefficient:λ, ant the training epochs T.

Output: Clustering results

1: Initialize the parameters of the network

2: **while** $epoch \leq T$ **do**

3: Feed **X** into multi-view construction module to get the multi-view data $\{X^p\}_{p=1}^{P}$.

4: Construct graph using Eq. (3.3)

5: Using graph convolution by to get the features Z^p Eq. (3.4)

6: Using multi-view contrastive learning to get the deep features by Eq. (3.9)

7: Undate parameters of the network by miniziming Eq. (3.10)

8: **end while**

9: Perform graph convolutional subspace clustering process to get the cluster labels

3.4 Experiments

To evaluate our model's performance, we conduct comprehensive clustering experiments across four established benchmark datasets, comparing against multiple cutting-edge clustering methods. The experimental configuration and detailed outcomes are systematically analyzed in subsequent sections.

3.4.1 Experiment's Setup

(1) Dataset: To ensure a rigorous evaluation of the model's performance, we utilize multiple established hyperspectral imaging datasets representing diverse scenarios. Our experimental validation incorporates four benchmark datasets: Indian Pines (AVIRIS sensor), Pavia University (ROSIS), Houston-2013 (ITRES CASI-1500), and Xu Zhou (HySpex). For practical implementation considerations, we worked with carefully chosen sub-regions from these scenes, with specific spatial extents documented in Table 3.2.

Indian Pines: The hyperspectral imagery under examination was captured by NASA's AVIRIS instrument over the Indian Pines test site. Our analysis focuses on a specific region spanning pixels [24–115], which contains 200 spectral channels for each pixel. With a ground sampling distance of 20 m, this subset represents four unique land cover categories.

Table 3.2 Statistics of the datasets used in our experiments

Dataset	Indian Pines	Pavia University	Houston	Xu Zhou
Pixels	85 × 70	200 × 100	349 × 680	100 × 260
Abscissa	30–115	150–350	0–349	0–100
Ordinate	24–94	100–200	0–680	0–260
Channels	200	103	144	436
Samples	4391	6445	6048	12,043
Clusters	4	8	12	5

Pavia University: The hyperspectral data was collected in 2003 using Germany's ROSIS imaging spectrometer, featuring high spatial resolution (1.3 m/pixel) and broad spectral coverage (430–860 nm) across 115 channels. Following quality control procedures that eliminated 12 bands affected by noise, we retained 103 spectral bands for subsequent analysis. Our study concentrated on a representative subregion defined by pixel coordinates [150–350, 100–200].

Houston 2013: The hyperspectral data was acquired in 2013 over Houston, Texas and surrounding rural regions using the ITRES CASI-1500 airborne sensor. Following preprocessing to remove noisy spectral channels, we utilized the remaining 144 high-quality bands for experimental validation. This dataset features a spatial resolution of 2.5 m per pixel and includes 12 distinct land cover classes—including vegetation types (trees, healthy grass), natural features (soil, water), and man-made surfaces (tennis courts, running tracks). Our analysis focused on a representative study area spanning pixel coordinates [0–349, 0–680].

Xu Zhou: The hyperspectral imagery was captured over a mining-affected suburban region of Xuzhou City in China's Jiangsu Province. Acquired by an airborne HySpex imaging spectrometer, the dataset exhibits exceptional spatial resolution (0.73 m/pixel) and broad spectral coverage (415–2508 nm) across 436 channels. For our analysis, we examined a representative subset [0–100, 0–260] containing five distinct surface types: agricultural fields, exposed soil, red-tiled roofs, vegetation canopies, and concrete surfaces (Table 3.3).

(2) Evaluation Metrics: For comprehensive performance evaluation of our proposed algorithm versus comparative methods, we employ three established quantitative metrics: Overall Accuracy (OA) for clustering precision, Normalized

Table 3.3 Important hyperparameters settings in our experiments

Dataset	Indian Pines	Pavia University	Houston	Xu Zhou
w	11	11	11	7
k	25	30	25	35
λ	100	1000	1000	100

Mutual Information (NMI) for cluster-label consistency, and Kappa coefficient (Kappa) for classification agreement analysis. These rigorously validated measures enable systematic comparison of algorithmic effectiveness, with detailed methodological explanations provided in the subsequent section.

1. OA is one of the most widely used clustering evaluation metrics. This refers to the proportion of correctly predicted samples among all samples. The formula for calculating the OA is as follows:

$$\mathrm{OA} = \frac{\sum_{1}^{N} \delta(y_i, \mathrm{map}(c_i))}{N}, \tag{3.14}$$

where N is the total number of samples, y_i represents the true label of data sample x_i, and c_i represents the predicted label of the algorithm. $\delta(\cdot)$ represents the indicator function, and its value is 1 if $y_i = \mathrm{map}(c_i)$; otherwise, its value is 0. $\mathrm{map}(\cdot)$ represents the mapping function, which rearranges the obtained labels to create the best match of the true labels.

2. NMI is an index used to measure the similarity between two clustering results:

$$\mathrm{NMI} = \frac{I(y_i, c_i)}{\sqrt{H(y_i)H(c_i)}}, \tag{3.15}$$

where $I(y_i, c_i)$ represents the mutual information between true and predicted labels. The larger value of $I(y_i, c_i)$ represents the closer the relationship between y_i and c_i. $H(\cdot)$ represents information entropy, which is the average amount of information corresponding to the entire probability distribution. The denominator in the formula is used to normalize the mutual information within the range [0,1].

3. Kappa is defined as:

$$\mathrm{Kappa} = \frac{N \sum_{i=1}^{m} h_{ii} - \sum_{i=1}^{m} (h_{i+} h_{+i})}{N^2 - \sum_{i=1}^{m} (h_{i+} h_{+i})}, \tag{3.16}$$

where h_{ii} represents the count of samples correctly classified into category i, and m represents the total number of categories. h_{i+} represents the total number of samples of the i-th category, and h_{+i} represents the number of samples classified as i-th. N is the total number of class samples.

3.4.2 Baseline

This study evaluates the performance of our novel model against established baseline approaches. The comparison includes two traditional clustering techniques—Spectral Clustering (SC) and Sparse Subspace Clustering (SSC), and alongside multiple state-of-the-art clustering methods introduced in recent literature.

- ***k*-means** [17] serves as a prominent example of classical unsupervised learning techniques.
  - **CL-CNN** employs contrastive learning alongside a convolutional neural network (CNN) to extract features, followed by clustering via k-means.
  - **SSC** [26] preserves subspace relationships by applying sparse regularization constraints.
- **l_2-SSC** [28] incorporates the l_2-norm while accounting for broader spatial dependencies.
  - **EGCSC** [36] pioneers the use of graph convolutional networks for HSI subspace clustering.
  - **RMMF** [52] fuses spectral-spatial data within a non-negative matrix factorization (NMF) framework to derive affinity matrices.
  - **NMFAML** [70] similarly leverages HSI spectral-spatial features through NMF for affinity matrix construction.
  - **GCOT** [53] incorporates optimal transport theory into graph-based representation learning, enhancing affinity matrix derivation.
  - **GR-RSCNet** [35] utilizes a deep neural network with graph regularization for HSI subspace clustering.
  - **HMSC** [38] generates multi-view representations, combining both local and nonlocal spatial information across views.
  - **HGCSC** [37]implements multihop hypergraph convolution, modeling intra-class associations as hypergraph edges.

3.4.3 Quantitative Results

The clustering results of the CMSCGC framework and comparative models across the four datasets are presented in Table 3.4. In the majority of cases, our approach attained superior performance across all three evaluation criteria—overall accuracy (OA), normalized mutual information (NMI), and Kappa coefficient—demonstrating a substantial advantage over competing methods. Notably, on the Indian Pines, Houston, and Xu Zhou datasets, the proposed technique exhibited a 3–5% increase in OA relative to the runner-up model. Additionally, several key patterns emerged from the analysis.

(1) The integration of deep learning techniques and regularization mechanisms has substantially enhanced clustering precision. Modern approaches leveraging neural networks, including GR-RSCNet, demonstrate notable advancements over conventional methods, underscoring the advantage of nonlinear transformations in deriving optimal feature representations for intricate real-world data clustering. The limited efficacy of CL-CNN stems from its reliance on the k-means algorithm, which lacks the precision of subspace clustering techniques. Additionally, conventional CNN-based feature extraction inadequately

Table 3.4 Clustering results (OA/NMI/KAPPA) of various methods on four benchmark datasets

Dataset	Metric	*k*-means	CL-CNN	SSC	l_2-SSC	RMMF	NMFAML	EGCSC	GCOT	HMSC	HGCSC	GR-RSCNet	CMSCGC
InP	OA	0.5953	0.6006	0.6558	0.6645	0.7121	0.8508	0.8483	0.8404	0.8901	0.9244	0.9317	**0.9761**
	NMI	0.4483	0.3288	0.6025	0.5382	0.4985	0.7264	0.6442	0.7654	0.8600	0.8921	0.8241	**0.9234**
	Kappa	0.4404	0.4057	0.5528	0.5263	0.5609	0.7809	0.6422	0.6258	0.9000	0.8307	0.9008	**0.9657**
PaU	OA	0.6027	0.6283	0.6548	0.6912	0.7704	0.8967	0.8442	0.9102	0.9482	0.9531	**0.9773**	0.9669
	NMI	0.5245	0.5901	0.6706	0.6251	0.7388	0.9216	0.8401	0.8804	0.9200	0.9383	0.9689	**0.9702**
	Kappa	0.6791	0.5706	0.5736	0.6881	0.6804	0.8625	0.7968	0.9233	0.8300	0.9440	**0.9702**	0.9565
Hou	OA	0.3932	0.4045	0.4581	0.5097	0.7309	0.6346	0.6238	0.6584	–	0.7315	0.8399	**0.8721**
	NMI	0.4101	0.3536	0.4961	0.5816	0.7797	0.7959	0.7754	0.7729	–	0.7004	0.8731	**0.9168**
	Kappa	0.3289	0.4281	0.4013	0.4811	0.6111	0.5917	0.5812	0.6167	–	0.8309	0.8221	**0.8584**
XuZ	OA	0.5778	0.6147	0.6638	0.6838	0.6111	0.8178	0.7834	0.8235	–	0.9157	0.9192	**0.9765**
	NMI	0.4049	0.5059	0.5357	0.5969	0.6253	0.7919	0.6975	0.6871	–	0.8862	0.8739	**0.9272**
	Kappa	0.4175	0.5155	0.4767	0.6592	0.4361	0.7459	0.6470	0.7620	–	0.8470	0.8649	**0.9681**

The best and suboptimal results are shown in bold and underlined, respectively preserves spatial relationships, compromising the discriminative power of the learned features. Among traditional approaches, l_2-SSC incorporates l_2-norm regularization, boosting accuracy by 10% on the Indian Pines dataset relative to standard SSC. Similarly, EGCSC employs graph regularization, while our proposed framework integrates contrastive learning regularization—both yielding substantial performance gains.

(2) The integration of multi-view complementary data significantly enhanced clustering performance. Among the benchmarked approaches, NMFAML also leverages homogeneous features to enrich representation learning. In a similar manner, our framework fuses spectral-textural attributes and employs a graph convolutional network (GCN) to effectively aggregate local structural patterns, substantially boosting clustering precision. Experimental results demonstrate accuracies of 97.61% (Indian Pines), 96.69% (Pavia University), 87.21% (Houston 2013), and 97.65% (Xu Zhou), validating the efficacy of our approach.

(3) The proposed CMSCGC framework demonstrated superior performance compared to EGCSC across all four benchmark datasets, achieving significant accuracy gains of 12.48%, 11.87%, 24.83%, and 19.31% respectively. These substantial improvements validate the effectiveness of three key innovations: multi-view data integration, contrastive learning-based regularization, and attention-based feature fusion mechanisms. The results establish CMSCGC as a novel and effective solution for hyperspectral image clustering tasks.

3.4.4 Qualitative Comparison of Different Methods

The clustering outcomes of different approaches on the four datasets (Indian Pines, Pavia University, Houston2013, and Xu Zhou) are visually presented in Figs. 3.2, 3.3, 3.4 and 3.5. Each figure's part (a) displays the ground reference data after background removal. It should be noted that while spectral clustering's unsupervised nature leads to inconsistent color assignments across methods for identical classes, this variation does not impact the comparative analysis. Current subspace clustering techniques exhibit notable limitations: while capable of dimensionality reduction for high-dimensional hyperspectral data, they fail to incorporate spatial relationships. Furthermore, conventional subspace clustering approaches demonstrate inadequate capability in effectively representing hyperspectral image structures, resulting in performance that falls short of modern deep learning alternatives (Figs. 3.6 and 3.7).

The proposed CMSCGC framework demonstrates superior visualization performance across all evaluated datasets. By adaptively integrating textural features, our approach significantly reduces speckle noise in the classified outputs compared to alternative methods. The graph convolutional network component enhances spatial consistency by effectively propagating neighborhood information, resulting in both improved intra-class uniformity and better preservation of object boundaries.

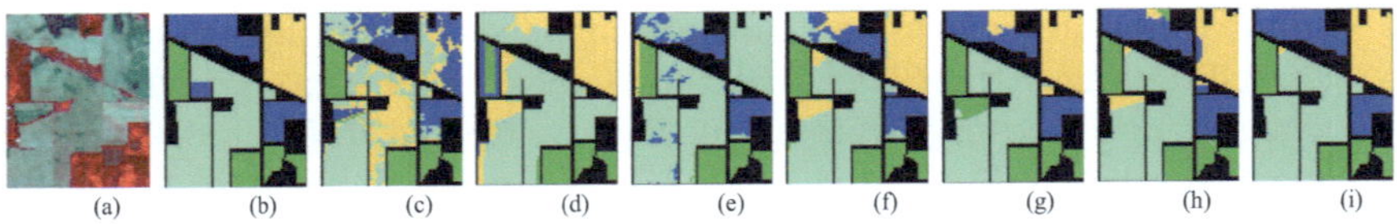

Fig. 3.2 Cluster visualization on the Indian Pines dataset: **b** false-color image **b** ground truth, **c** k-means, **d** SSC, **e** l2-SSC, **f** EGCSC, **g** HGCSC, **h** GR-RSCNet, and **i** our proposed CMSCGC

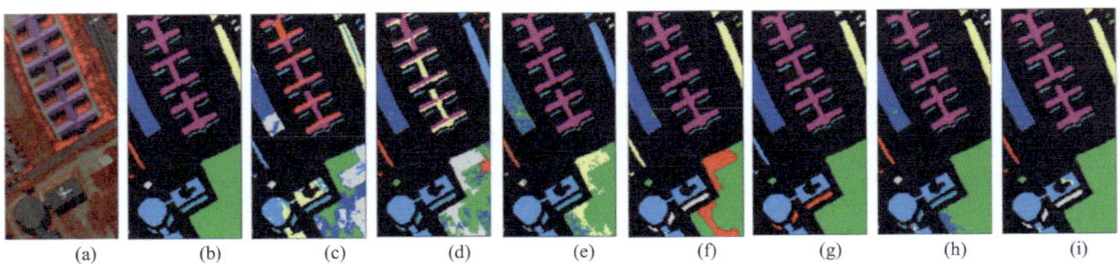

Fig. 3.3 Cluster visualization on the Pavia University dataset: **b** false-color image **b** ground truth, **c** k-means, **d** SSC, **e** l2-SSC, **f** EGCSC, **g** HGCSC, **h** GR-RSCNet, and **i** our proposed CMSCGC

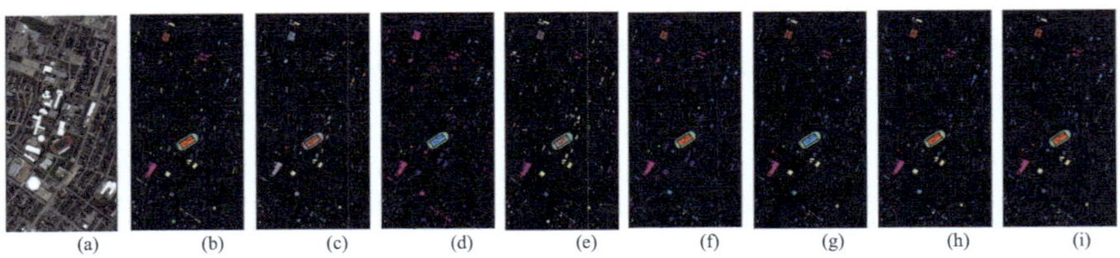

Fig. 3.4 Cluster visualization on the Houston-2013 dataset: **b** false-color image **b** ground truth, **c** k-means, **d** SSC, **e** l2-SSC, **f** EGCSC, **g** HGCSC, **h** GR-RSCNet, and **i** our proposed CMSCGC

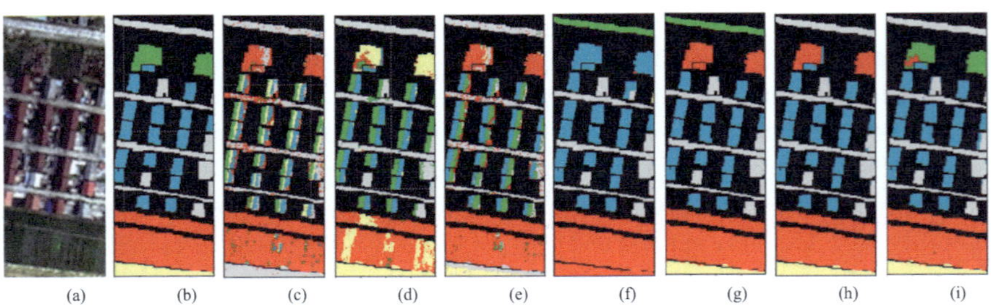

Fig. 3.5 Cluster visualization on the Xu Zhou dataset: **b** false-color image **b** ground truth, **c** k-means, **d** SSC, **e** l2-SSC, **f** EGCSC, **g** HGCSC, **h** GR-RSCNet, and **i** our proposed CMSCGC

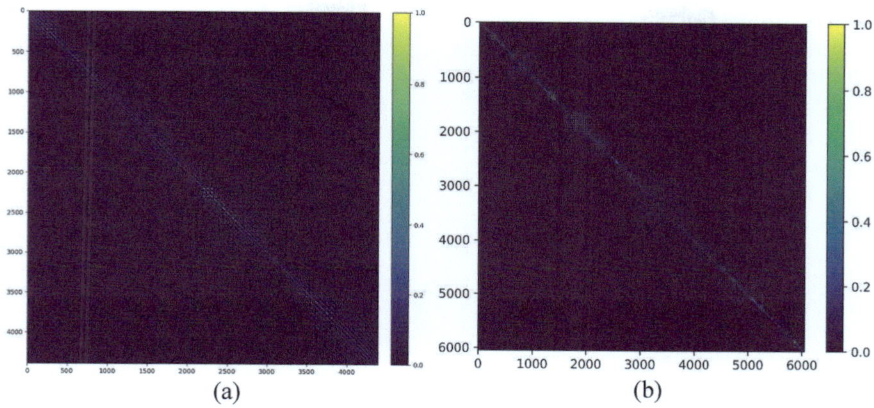

Fig. 3.6 Visualization of the affinity matrix learn on **b** Indian Pines. **b** Houston

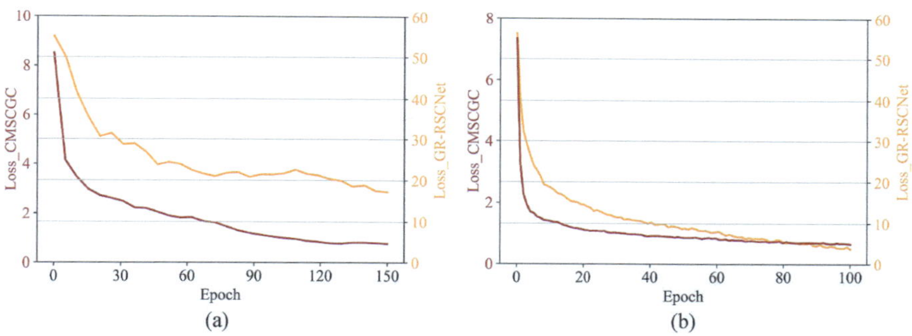

Fig. 3.7 Loss curves of the CMSCGC and GR-RSCNet. **b** Indian Pines. **b** Pavia University

3.4.5 Parameter Analysis

Our research systematically examines the influence of three key hyperparameters on the CMSCGC framework's performance. The optimal parameter configurations employed in our experimental evaluation are detailed in Table 3.3.

Sensitivity to regularization coefficient λ: The regularization parameter λ was evaluated across a logarithmic scale ($S = \{0.01, 0.1, 1, 10, 100, 1000\}$), with the comprehensive performance analysis presented in Fig. 3.8. For the Houston dataset, we observed that smaller λ values consistently led to degraded performance across all evaluation metrics (OA, NMI, and Kappa). This phenomenon likely occurs because the Houston dataset's characteristic dispersed spectral distribution requires stronger regularization to maintain meaningful connectivity in the learned structural affinity matrix during spectral embedding. In contrast, the Xu Zhou dataset exhibited remarkable stability, with our method achieving near-optimal performance across a wide

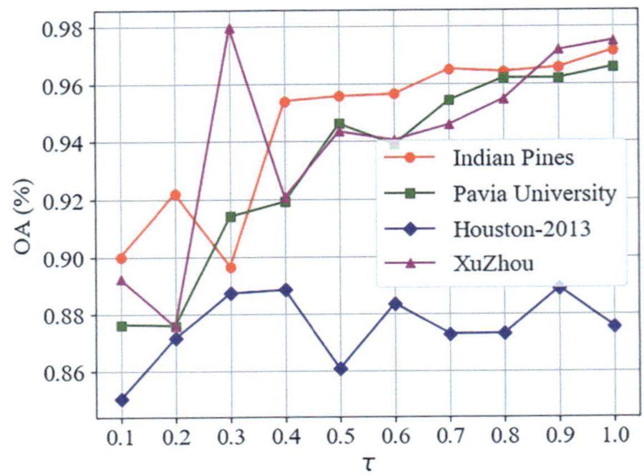

Fig. 3.8 Performance comparison on four datasets with different regularization coefficient λ

range of λ values. This demonstrates the framework's inherent robustness to parameter variations while maintaining high clustering accuracy, as evidenced by consistent results for all three evaluation metrics throughout the tested parameter spectrum.

Sensitivity to nearest neighbors k**:** The construction of graph embeddings for hyperspectral imagery relies on selecting an appropriate number of nearest neighbors (k) in the k-NN graph. To systematically evaluate this parameter's influence, we conducted experiments with k values ranging from 20 to 40 in increments of 5 while maintaining fixed values for other hyperparameters. Figure 3.9 reveals a consistent performance degradation across all three evaluation metrics when k exceeds optimal values, primarily attributed to the over-smoothing effect caused by excessive neighborhood aggregation. Based on these findings, we established dataset-specific optimal k values: 25 for Indian Pines, 30 for Pavia University, 25 for Houston 2013, and 35 for Xu Zhou, ensuring balanced neighborhood information incorporation without compromising feature discrimination.

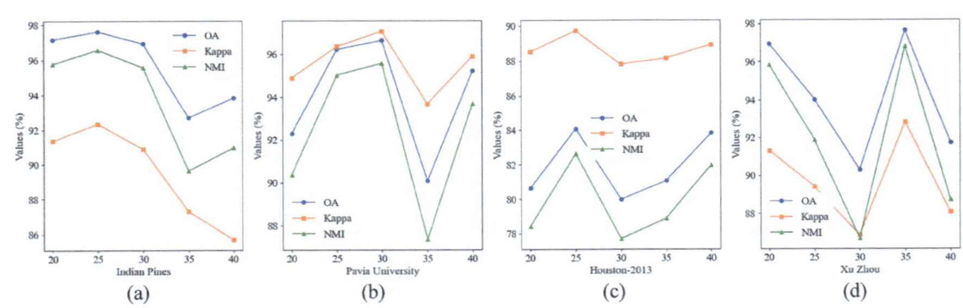

Fig. 3.9 Performance comparison on four datasets with different number of neighbors k. **a** Indian Pines dataset. **b** Pavia University dataset. **c** Houston-2013 dataset. **d** Xu Zhou dataset

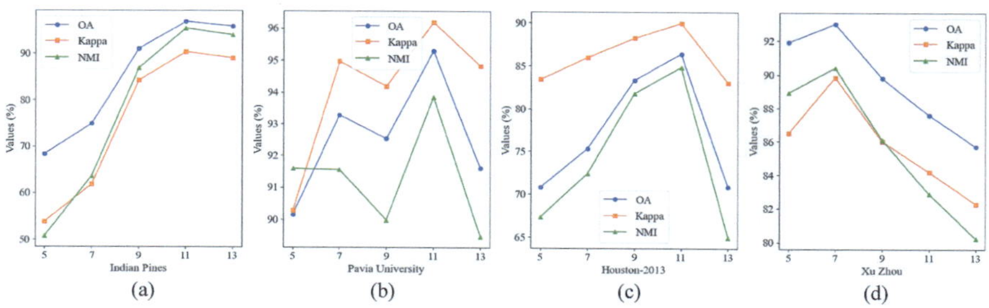

Fig. 3.10 Performance comparison on four datasets with different input size w. **a** Indian Pines dataset. **b** Pavia University dataset. **c** Houston-2013 dataset. **d** Xu Zhou dataset

3.4.6 Ablation Experiments

To validate the architectural design of our network, we performed comprehensive ablation studies to assess the individual contributions of each module. The quantitative evaluation, presented in Table 3.5, demonstrates the model's performance across four benchmark datasets: Indian Pines, Pavia University, Houston 2013, and Xu Zhou. These results represent averaged metrics from 10 independent experimental trials, providing statistically reliable evidence for the structural efficacy of each network component.

(1) **Ablation Study on Multi-View Fusion:** While prior findings confirm that integrating multi-view data enhances clustering performance, we further validate this through a comparative analysis of single-view (spectral or textural) and multi-view approaches (Table 3.5). The single-view outcomes are suboptimal, whereas multi-view fusion yields substantial accuracy gains. Notably, while the textural view alone does not outperform the spatial-spectral view, the combined multi-view method achieves improvements of 7.68%, 2.85%, 18.56%, and 10.61% on the Indian Pines, Pavia University, Houston-2013, and Xu Zhou datasets, respectively. This demonstrates that textural features effectively supplement spatial-spectral data, enabling better extraction of land-cover

Table 3.5 Ablation studies (OA) for different views, contrastive learning, and attention fusion module for CMSCGC

No.	Texture features	Spectral-spatial features	Contrastive learning	Attention fusion	InP	PaU	Hou	XuZ
1	√	×	×	×	0.6961	0.8479	0.6096	0.7678
2	×	√	×	×	0.8483	0.8442	0.6238	0.7834
3	√	√	×	×	0.9251	0.8727	0.8094	0.8895
4	√	√	√	×	0.9541	0.9103	0.8545	0.9504
5	√	√	√	√	**0.9761**	**0.9669**	**0.8721**	**0.9765**

The best and suboptimal results are shown in bold and underline, respectively spatial patterns. Consequently, their synergistic integration leads to superior clustering results.

(2) **Ablation study on contrastive learning:** Table 3.5 presents a comparison between models trained with and without contrastive learning loss (Cases 3 and Cases 4). The results demonstrate that incorporating contrastive learning consistently enhances performance across all datasets, yielding superior overall accuracy (OA), normalized mutual information (NMI), and Kappa coefficient. Specifically, the inclusion of contrastive learning led to accuracy improvements of 2.9%, 3.76%, 4.51%, and 6.09% on the respective datasets. These findings underscore the critical role of contrastive loss in boosting clustering effectiveness.

(3) **Ablation study on adaptive affinity matrix:** Table 3.5 compares two variants of our model: Case 5, which employs a basic averaging approach for affinity matrix fusion, and Case 4, which incorporates an attention-based adaptive fusion module. The results demonstrate that the attention-driven fusion strategy consistently outperforms simple averaging, achieving accuracy gains of 2.2%, 5.66%, 1.76%, and 2.61% across the four datasets. This improvement confirms that dynamically weighting multi-view feature representations through attention mechanisms enhances hyperspectral image (HSI) clustering performance compared to static fusion methods.

To further validate our approach, we compared the learned affinity matrices on the Indian Pines dataset, as illustrated in Fig. 3.6. The visualization reveals that CMSCGC produces a sparser and more distinct block-diagonal structure compared to baseline methods. This enhanced structure suggests improved discrimination of intra-class similarities, demonstrating the model's ability to effectively capture underlying cluster relationships. The observed improvements stem from the adaptive fusion of textural and spectral features, which refines feature representation and contributes to more precise hyperspectral image classification.

3.4.7 Running Time Comparison

Table 3.6 compares the runtime performance between conventional shallow clustering approaches (SSC, EGCSC, GCOT, HGCSC) and contemporary deep learning methods (CL-CNN, GR-RSCNet, CMSCGC), with all experiments conducted on identical GPU hardware. The results reveal a clear trade-off between computational speed and feature quality: shallow methods demonstrate faster execution by operating directly on extracted features, while deep approaches require iterative training to learn more discriminative representations. Among deep methods, CMSCGC shows superior computational efficiency compared to GR-SCNet, demonstrating that our GR-RSCNet framework successfully optimizes the performance-efficiency balance.

Table 3.6 Running time of different methods (in second)

Method	InP	PaU	Hou	XuZ
CL-CNN	873.9	1520.1	3534.7	13,619.6
SSC	226.5	439.3	907	657.3
EGCSC	23.9	53.3	55.5	201.4
GCOT	21.6	64.1	121.4	209.2
HGCSC	54	204.9	9353.1	421.3
GR-RSCNet	3282.6	10,134.7	14,876	6077.6
CMSCGC	96.1	614.5	3269.1	754.2

Table 3.7 Clustering performance of different views for the Indian pine dataset

No.	View	OA	NMI	Kappa
1	HSI + EMP	0.9761	0.9234	0.9567
2	HSI + Gabor	0.9604	0.9163	0.9486
3	HSI + Gabor + EMP	0.9832	0.9329	0.9585

This efficiency advantage, combined with CMSCGC's enhanced clustering accuracy (demonstrated in previous sections), positions it as a practical solution for hyperspectral image analysis.

3.4.8 Clustering with Different Views

To demonstrate the effectiveness of CMSCGC in multi-view learning, Table 3.7 displays clustering outcomes for the Indian Pines dataset across distinct feature representations. The term "HSI" refers to the image's inherent spectral-spatial characteristics, while "EMP" and "Gabor" signify additional perspectives derived from EMP-based and 2-D Gabor filter-based feature extraction methods, respectively. The findings reveal that incorporating all three views improves overall accuracy (OA) by 0.71% and 2.28%, respectively, over models utilizing only two views. These results highlight the model's proficiency in integrating multi-view data while emphasizing the synergistic benefits of diverse feature sets in clustering performance.

3.4.9 Clustering with Different Loss Functions

Modern clustering techniques can be broadly classified into two dominant paradigms: contrastive clustering and reconstructive clustering. Contrastive approaches are

Table 3.8 Clustering performance of different loss functions for the Indian pine dataset

Method	InP	PaU	Hou	XuZ
MSCGC	0.9251	0.8727	0.8094	0.8895
CMSCGC w/o NS	0.9317	0.9025	0.7947	0.9036
MSCGC w BT	0.9334	0.9361	0.8054	0.9277
MSCGC w RC	0.9589	0.9434	0.8375	0.9491
CMSCGC	0.9761	0.9669	0.8721	0.9765

further subdivided based on whether they incorporate negative samples. To evaluate clustering performance, we analyze several methodologies: lossless multi-view subspace clustering using graph convolutional networks (MSCGC), contrastive clustering without negative samples (CMSCGC without NS), reconstructive clustering (MSCGC without RC), and conventional contrastive clustering (CMSCGC). These methods primarily rely on sample-level contrastive learning. Additionally, we develop feature-level comparative frameworks by integrating the baseline MSCGC model with Barlow Twins loss (MSCGC with BT). As evidenced in Table 3.8, CMSCGC achieves superior performance, whereas reconstructive clustering underperforms. This disparity stems from MSCGC's reliance on shallow feature extraction without feature optimization. The MSCGC with BT variant struggles with inter-class differentiation, leading to diminished results. Similarly, CMSCGC without NS exhibits reduced clustering efficacy due to the exclusion of negative samples, which hinders precise inter-cluster separation.

3.5 Conclusion

This chapter introduces CMSCGC, an innovative multi-view subspace clustering framework designed for hyperspectral image analysis. The proposed methodology begins by deriving both textural and spectral features from HSIs to establish a multi-view graph representation. Graph convolutional networks are subsequently employed to integrate local neighborhood characteristics, while contrastive learning simultaneously captures consistent and complementary patterns across views. The resulting enhanced features serve as input to a self-expression module for affinity matrix generation. To address the varying importance of different feature perspectives, an attention mechanism dynamically weights the contributions of each view during the fusion process, yielding more discriminative affinity representations. The framework's effectiveness is validated through extensive experiments on four benchmark hyperspectral datasets, where it demonstrates superior performance compared to existing state-of-the-art methods. Additional ablation studies systematically confirm the individual contributions of each architectural component to the overall clustering improvement.

The self-expression layer in the current architecture presents scalability limitations when applied to large-scale datasets. While mini-batch processing partially mitigates computational constraints, this approach inherently restricts the graph convolutional networks' capacity to capture comprehensive relational patterns. Future work will focus on enhancing CMSCGC's scalability to better leverage its potential on extensive datasets.

References

1. Camps-Valls G, Tuia D, Bruzzone L, Benediktsson JA (2013) Advances in hyperspectral image classification: earth monitoring with statistical learning methods. IEEE Signal Process Mag 31(1):45–54
2. Zhao Y-P, Li H, Chen Y, Wang Z, Li X (2023) Hyperspectral anomaly detection via structured sparsity plus enhanced low-rankness. IEEE Trans Geosci Rem Sens 61:1–15
3. Guan R, Li Z, Li T, Li X, Yang J, Chen W (2022) Classification of heterogeneous mining areas based on rescapsnet and gaofen-5 imagery. Remote Sensing 14(13):3216
4. Chen Y, Yuan Q, Tang Y, Xiao Y, He J, Zhang L (2023) Spirit: spectral awareness interaction network with dynamic template for hyperspectral object tracking. IEEE Trans Geosci Rem Sens 62:1–16
5. Tang Y, Feng S, Zhao C, Fan Y, Shi Q, Li W, Tao R (2024) An object fine-grained change detection method based on frequency decoupling interaction for high-resolution remote sensing images. IEEE Trans Geosci Remote Sens 62:1–13
6. Zhao C, Qin B, Feng S, Zhu W, Sun W, Li W, Jia X (2023) Hyperspectral image classification with multi-attention transformer and adaptive superpixel segmentation-based active learning. IEEE Trans Image Process 32:3606–3621
7. Chen Y, Tang Y, Yin Z, Han T, Zou B, Feng H (2022) Single object tracking in satellite videos: a correlation filter-based dual-flow tracker. IEEE J Select Top Appl Earth Observ Remote Sens 15:6687–6698
8. Chen W, Ouyang S, Yang J, Li X, Zhou G, Wang L (2022) Jagan: A framework for complex land cover classification using gaofen-5 AHSI images. IEEE J Select Top Appl Earth Observ Remote Sens 15:1591–1603
9. Liu J, Guan R, Li Z, Zhang J, Hu Y, Wang X (2023) Adaptive multi-feature fusion graph convolutional network for hyperspectral image classification. Remote Sens 15(23):5483
10. Tarabalka Y, Fauvel M, Chanussot J, Benediktsson JA (2010) Svm-and mrf-based method for accurate classification of hyperspectral images. IEEE Geosci Remote Sens Lett 7(4):736–740
11. Chen Y, Lin Z, Zhao X, Wang G, Gu Y (2014) Deep learning-based classification of hyperspectral data. IEEE J Select Top Appl Earth Observ Remote Sens 7(6):2094–2107
12. Wang R, Nie F, Yu W (2017) Fast spectral clustering with anchor graph for large hyperspectral images. IEEE Geosci Remote Sens Lett 14(11):2003–2007
13. Zhai H, Zhang H, Li P, Zhang L (2021) Hyperspectral image clustering: current achievements and future lines. IEEE Geosci Rem Sens Mag 9(4):35–67
14. Hu D, Liang K, Zhou S, Tu W, Liu M, Liu X (2023) SCDFC: a deep fusion clustering method for single-cell RNA-SEQ data. Brief Bioinform bbad216
15. Borsoi RA, Imbiriba T, Bermudez JCM, Richard C, Chanussot J, Drumetz L, Tourneret J-Y, Zare A, Jutten C (2021) Spectral variability in hyperspectral data unmixing: a comprehensive review. IEEE Geosci Rem Sens Mag 9(4):223–270
16. Chang J, Meng G, Wang L, Xiang S, Pan C (2018) Deep self-evolution clustering. IEEE Trans Pattern Anal Mach Intell 42(4):809–823
17. Kanungo T, Mount DM, Netanyahu NS, Piatko CD, Silverman R, Wu AY (2002) An efficient k-means clustering algorithm: analysis and implementation. IEEE Trans Pattern Anal Mach Intell 24(7):881–892

18. Ghaffarian S, Ghaffarian S (2014) Automatic histogram-based fuzzy c-means clustering for remote sensing imagery. ISPRS J Photogramm Remote Sens 97:46–57
19. Comaniciu D, Meer P (2002) Mean shift: a robust approach toward feature space analysis. IEEE Trans Pattern Anal Mach Intell 24(5):603–619
20. Chen Y, Ma S, Chen X, Ghamisi P (2017) Hyperspectral data clustering based on density analysis ensemble. Remote sensing letters 8(2):194–203
21. Vidal R (2011) Subspace clustering. IEEE Signal Process Mag 28(2):52–68
22. Liu S, Wang S, Zhang P, Xu K, Liu X, Zhang C, Gao F (2022) Effi- cient one-pass multi-view subspace clustering with consensus anchors. Proc AAAI Conf Artif Intell 36(7):7576–7584
23. Liu S, Liu X, Wang S, Niu X, Zhu E (2022) Fast incomplete multi-view clustering with view-independent anchors. IEEE Trans Neural Netw Learn Syst
24. Ou Q, Wang S, Zhou S, Li M, Guo X, Zhu E (2020) Anchor-based multiview subspace clustering with diversity regularization. IEEE Multimedia 27(4):91–101
25. Li Q, Liu W, Li L (2018) Affinity learning via a diffusion process for subspace clustering. Pattern Recogn 84:39–50
26. Zhang H, Zhai H, Zhang L, Li P (2016) Spectral–spatial sparse subspace clustering for hyperspectral remote sensing images. IEEE Trans Geosci Remote Sens 54(6):3672–3684
27. Vidal R, Favaro P (2014) Low rank subspace clustering (lrsc). Pattern Recogn Lett 43:47–61
28. Zhai H, Zhang H, Zhang L, Li P, Plaza A (2016) A new sparse sub-space clustering algorithm for hyperspectral remote sensing imagery. IEEE Geosci Remote Sens Lett 14(1):43–47
29. Huang S, Zhang H, Piˇzurica A (2019) Semisupervised sparse subspace clustering method with a joint sparsity constraint for hyperspectral remote sensing images. IEEE J Select Top Appl Earth Observ Remote Sens 12(3):989–999
30. Tu W, Guan R, Zhou S, Ma C, Peng X, Cai Z, Liu Z, Cheng J, Liu X (2024) Attribute-missing graph clustering network
31. Peng Z, Liu H, Jia Y, Hou J (2022) Adaptive attribute and structure subspace clustering network. IEEE Trans Image Process 31:3430–3439
32. Liu M, Liu Y, Liang K, Wang S, Zhou S, Liu X (2023) Deep temporalgraph clustering. arXiv preprint arXiv:2305.10738
33. Lei J, Li X, Peng B, Fang L, Ling N, Huang Q (2020) Deep spatial-spectral subspace clustering for hyperspectral image. IEEE Trans Circuits Syst Video Technol 31(7):2686–2697
34. Li K, Qin Y, Ling Q, Wang Y, Lin Z, An W (2021) Self-supervised deep subspace clustering for hyperspectral images with adaptive self-expressive coefficient matrix initialization. IEEE J Select Top Appl Earth Observ Remote Sens 14:3215–3227
35. Cai Y, Zeng M, Cai Z, Liu X, Zhang Z (2021) Graph regularized residual subspace clustering network for hyperspectral image clustering. Inf Sci 578:85–101
36. Cai Y, Zhang Z, Cai Z, Liu X, Jiang X, Yan Q (2020) Graph convolutional subspace clustering: A robust subspace clustering framework for hyperspectral image. IEEE Trans Geosci Remote Sens 59(5):4191–4202
37. Zhang Z, Cai Y, Gong W, Ghamisi P, Liu X, Gloaguen R (2021) Hypergraph convolutional subspace clustering with multihop aggregation for hyperspectral image. IEEE J Select Top Appl Earth Observ Remote Sens 15:676–686
38. Huang S, Zhang H, Piˇzurica A (2021) Hybrid-hypergraph regularized multiview subspace clustering for hyperspectral images. IEEE Trans Geosci Remote Sens 60:1–16
39. Hinojosa C, Rojas F, Castillo S, Arguello H (2021) Hyperspectral image segmentation using 3d regularized subspace clustering model. J Appl Rem Sens 15(1):016508–016508
40. Benediktsson JA, Palmason JA, Sveinsson JR (2005) Classification of hyperspectral data from urban areas based on extended morphological profiles. IEEE Trans Geosci Remote Sens 43(3):480–491
41. Li W, Chen C, Su H, Du Q (2015) Local binary patterns and extreme learning machine for hyperspectral imagery classification. IEEE Trans Geosci Remote Sens 53(7):3681–3693
42. Wang J, Tang C, Wan Z, Zhang W, Sun K, Zomaya AY (2023) Efficient and effective one-step multiview clustering. IEEE Trans Neural Netw Learn Syst

43. Tian L, Du Q, Kopriva I, Younan N (2018) Spatial-spectral based multi-view low-rank sparse sbuspace clustering for hyperspectral imagery. In:IGARSS 2018—2018 IEEE international geoscience and remote sensing symposium. IEEE, pp 8488–8491
44. Chen Z, Zhang C, Mu T, He Y (2022) Tensorial multiview subspace clustering for polarimetric hyperspectral images. IEEE Trans Geosci Remote Sens 60:1–13
45. Lu H, Su H, Hu J, Du Q (2022) Dynamic ensemble learning with multi-view kernel collaborative subspace clustering for hyperspectral image classification. IEEE J Select Top Appl Earth Observ Remote Sens 15:2681–2695
46. Cai Y, Zhang Z, Ghamisi P, Ding Y, Liu X, Cai Z, Gloaguen R (2022) Superpixel contracted neighborhood contrastive subspace clustering network for hyperspectral images. IEEE Trans Geosci Remote Sens 60:1–13
47. Zhu Y, Xu Y, Yu F, Liu Q, Wu S, Wang L (2021) Graph contrastive learning with adaptive augmentation. Proc Web Conf 2021:2069–2080
48. Xie Y, Zhang W, Qu Y, Dai L, Tao D (2020) Hyper-laplacian regularized multilinear multiview self-representations for clustering and semisupervised learning. IEEE Trans Cybern 50(2):572–586
49. Hu D, Dong Z, Liang K, Wang J, Wang S, Liu X (2023) Single-cell multi-view clustering via community detection with unknown number of clusters. arXiv preprint arXiv:2311.17103
50. Chen Y, Wang S, Peng C, Hua Z, Zhou Y (2021) Generalized nonconvex low-rank tensor approximation for multi-view subspace clustering. IEEE Trans Image Process 30:4022–4035
51. Chen Y, Xiao X, Peng C, Lu G, Zhou Y (2021) Low-rank tensor graph learning for multi-view subspace clustering. IEEE Trans Circuits Syst Video Technol 32(1):92–104
52. Zhang L, Zhang L, Du B, You J, Tao D (2019) Hyperspectral image unsupervised classification by robust manifold matrix factorization. Inf Sci 485:154–169
53. Liu S, Wang H (2022) Graph convolutional optimal transport for hyperspectral image spectral clustering. IEEE Trans Geosci Remote Sens 60:1–13
54. Liu R (2021) Understand and improve contrastive learning methods for visualrepresentation: a review. arXiv preprint arXiv:2106.03259
55. Van Gansbeke W, Vandenhende S, Georgoulis S, Proesmans M, Van Gool L (2020) Scan: learning to classify images without labels. In:European conference on computer vision. Springer, pp 268– 285
56. Chen T, Kornblith S, Norouzi M, Hinton G (2020) A simple frameworkfor contrastive learning of visual representations. In: International conference on machine learning. PMLR, pp 1597–1607
57. He K, Fan H, Wu Y, Xie S, Girshick R (2020) Momentum contrastfor unsupervised visual representation learning. In: Proceedings of the IEEE/CVF conference on computer vision and pattern recognition, pp 9729–9738
58. Grill J-B, Strub F, Altche F, Tallec C, Richemond P, Buchatskaya E, Doersch C, Avila Pires B, Guo Z, Gheshlaghi Azar M et al (2020) Bootstrap your own latent-a new approach to self-supervised learning. Adv Neural Inform Proces Syst 33:21271–21284
59. Chen X, He K (2021) Exploring simple SIAMESE representation learning.In: Proceedings of the IEEE/CVF conference on computer vision and pattern recognition, pp 15750–15758
60. Zbontar J, Jing L, Misra I, LeCun Y, Deny S (2021) Barlow twins:self-supervised learning via redundancy reduction. In: International conference on machine learning. PMLR, pp 12310–12320
61. Liu Y, Tu W, Zhou S, Liu X, Song L, Yang X, Zhu E (2022) Deep graph clustering via dual correlation reduction. Proc AAAI Conf Artif Intell 36(7):7603–7611
62. Tu W, Zhou S, Liu X, Ge C, Cai Z, Liu Y (2023) Hierarchicallycontrastive hard sample mining for graph self-supervised pretraining. IEEE Trans Neural Netw Learn Syst 1–14
63. Guan R, Li Z, Li X, Tang C (2023) Pixel-superpixel contrastive learningand pseudo-label correction for hyperspectral image clustering. arXiv preprint arXiv:2312.09630
64. Hou S, Shi H, Cao X, Zhang X, Jiao L (2021) Hyperspectral imagery classification based on contrastive learning. IEEE Trans Geosci Remote Sens 60:1–13

65. Wang J-X, Li T, Chen S-B, Tang J, Luo B, Wilson RC (2022) Reliable contrastive learning for semi-supervised change detection in remote sensing images. IEEE Trans Geosci Remote Sens 60:1–13
66. Li H, Li Y, Zhang G, Liu R, Huang H, Zhu Q, Tao C (2022) Global and local contrastive self-supervised learning for semantic segmentation of hr remote sensing images. IEEE Trans Geosci Remote Sens 60:1–14
67. Wang M, Gao F, Dong J, Li H-C, Du Q (2023) Nearest neighbor- based contrastive learning for hyperspectral and Lidar data classification. IEEE Trans Geosci Remote Sens 61:1–16
68. Rodarmel C, Shan J (2002) Principal component analysis for hyperspectral image classification. Surv Land Inform Sci 62(2):115–122
69. Fauvel M, Tarabalka Y, Benediktsson JA, Chanussot J, Tilton JC (2012) Advances in spectral-spatial classification of hyperspectral images. Proc IEEE 101(3):652–675
70. Qin Y, Li B, Ni W, Quan S, Wang P, Bian H (2020) Affinity matrix learning via nonnegative matrix factorization for hyperspectral imagery clustering. IEEE J Select Top Appl Earth Observ Remote Sens 14:402–415
71. Liu Y, Xia J, Zhou S, Wang S, Guo X, Yang X, Liang K, Tu W, Li ZS, Liu X (2022) A survey of deep graph clustering: taxonomy,challenge, and application. arXiv preprint arXiv:2211.12875
72. Tian F, Gao B, Cui Q, Chen E, Liu T-Y (2014) Learning deep representations for graph clustering. Proc AAAI Conf Artif Intell 28(1)

Chapter 4
An Efficient Low-Pass Contrastive Graph Clustering Network for Hyperspectral Images

4.1 Introduction

Hyperspectral imaging (HSI), propelled by advancements in remote sensing (RS), has emerged as a powerful analytical tool across diverse domains such as environmental surveillance, geological analysis, target identification, and military operations, owing to its capacity to capture detailed spectral data [1]. A core task in HSI analysis involves categorizing each pixel into distinct classes, a process that has garnered substantial research interest [2, 3].

Contemporary approaches to HSI classification encompass both traditional machine learning techniques—including logistic regression [7], k-nearest neighbors [8], support vector machines [9], and random forests [10]—and advanced deep learning architectures like convolutional neural networks (CNNs) [11] and transformers [12]. These frameworks predominantly rely on supervised or semi-supervised paradigms, necessitating annotated training datasets that demand domain expertise and considerable manual effort [13, 14]. Additionally, such approaches inherently struggle to resolve data leakage issues, a persistent challenge in predictive modeling. In contrast, unsupervised methods like clustering have gained traction for their ability to operate without labeled data, though they require robust feature extraction capabilities to discern inherent patterns and spatial-spectral relationships in HSI [15, 16].

Clustering in HSI aims to group pixels of identical landcover categories by optimizing intra-class homogeneity and inter-class separation [17, 18]. Initial efforts employed conventional algorithms like k-means [20], fuzzy c-means (FCM) [21], and kernel-based fuzzy clustering [19], originally devised for natural imagery. However, these methods falter when handling HSI's spectral intricacy. Subspace clustering, which represents data points via linear combinations within shared subspaces [22], later addressed these limitations by integrating spatial-spectral features. Techniques such as sparse subspace clustering (SSC) [24] and its l2-norm variant [25] improved

Y. Ding et al., *Graph Neural Network for Hyperspectral Image Clustering*, Intelligent Perception and Information Processing, https://doi.org/10.1007/978-981-96-7710-8_4

clustering efficacy through affinity matrix optimization and neighborhood-aware coefficient constraints.

Despite progress, traditional methods exhibit constrained accuracy due to shallow feature representations. Deep clustering frameworks have thus emerged, leveraging nonlinear feature extraction. For instance, Zhao et al. [26] embedded regularized linear models into networks for structural feature learning, while Hu et al. [27] applied contrastive learning to spatial-spectral data. Graph-based models further advanced the field by exploiting relational structures among pixels. Cai et al. [28, 29] utilized graph-driven spectral clustering, whereas Wang et al. [30] incorporated anchor graphs to harness spectral-spatial attributes. Hypergraphs [31] and pixel-superpixel graphs [4] captured higher-order correlations, and contrastive frameworks [32] enhanced feature robustness through sample consistency. Ding et al. [33] employed autoencoder-based graph attention networks for large-scale HSI, yet noise sensitivity and computational overhead remain unresolved [34].

To overcome these challenges, this work proposes a self-supervised low-pass contrastive graph clustering framework (SLCGC) for HSI. The methodology begins with superpixel-based graph construction, followed by a low-pass denoising mechanism to suppress noise via neighborhood aggregation. Dual multilayer perceptrons (MLPs) then refine high-order spectral-spatial features, while Siamese encoders generate augmented views for contrastive learning. A novel cross-view loss enhances structural consistency, and K-means is applied to latent features for final clustering. The innovative contributions of our SLCGC are as follows:

- A novel denoising framework is introduced to eliminate high-frequency noise in graph structures while retaining smoothed node features through neighborhood information aggregation. This process enhances structural stability by prioritizing low-frequency signal preservation.
- Dual multilayer perceptrons (MLPs) are integrated to encode denoised graph features, augmented with Gaussian noise perturbations to generate dual-view representations. These contrasting perspectives enable robust feature learning for clustering tasks.
- An innovative contrastive loss function is formulated to align structural coherence across augmented views, strengthening the model's discriminative power and reducing feature redundancy.

We organize the rest of this chapter as follows: Sect. 4.2 presents a notations summary, graph filter, and contrastive learning in detail. Section 4.3 introduces the structure details of SLCGC for HSI clustering. Section 4.4 analyzes and describes the experimental results. Finally, the conclusion and further research are presented in Sect. 4.5.

Table 4.1 Main notions summery

Notation	Meaning
$\mathcal{G} = (V; E)$	Graph $\mathcal{G}$ with edge set E and node set V
N	Graph node number
$\boldsymbol{X} \in \mathbb{R}^{N \times D}$	Node feature matrix
$\boldsymbol{x}_i$	The i-th node feature
$\boldsymbol{A} \in \mathbb{R}^{N \times N}$	Adjacency matrix
S_i	The i th superpixel
n_i	The number of pixels contained in S_i
$\boldsymbol{Q} \in \mathbb{R}^{hw \times N}$	The correlation matrix
h, w, and b	The height, width, and number of bands of the HSI
$\hat{\boldsymbol{Q}}$	Normalized $\boldsymbol{Q}$
$\boldsymbol{H}$	Graph Laplacian filter
$\boldsymbol{L}, \tilde{\boldsymbol{L}}$	The graph Laplacian matrix and its symmetric normalized
$\boldsymbol{X}_t$	The smoothed node feature
$\boldsymbol{Z}^{l_1}$ and $\boldsymbol{Z}^{l_2}$	Two augmented views
$\boldsymbol{N} \in \mathbb{R}^{N \times d}$	Random Gaussian noise
$\boldsymbol{Z} \in \mathbb{R}^{N \times d}$	The clustering-oriented node features
$\boldsymbol{S} \in \mathbb{R}^{N \times N}$	The similarity matrix
$\hat{\mathbf{A}} = \boldsymbol{I} + \boldsymbol{A} \in \mathbb{R}^{N \times N}$	The self-looped adjacency matrix
$\mathcal{L}$	The cross-view contrastive loss

4.2 Related Concepts and Definition

4.2.1 Notations Summery

Given a node set $\mathcal{V} = \{v_1, v_2, \ldots, v_N\}$ with N nodes, C classes and edge set$\mathcal{E}$, an undirected graph $\mathcal{G} = \{\boldsymbol{X}, \boldsymbol{A}\}$ can be constructed, where $\boldsymbol{X} \in \mathbb{R}^{N \times D}$ and $\boldsymbol{A} \in \mathbb{R}^{N \times N}$ are the feature matrix and adjacency matrix of the constructed graph, respectively. We summery the notions in Table 4.1.

4.2.2 Graph Filter

In signal processing, the Fourier convolution operation for discrete signal $\hat{f}_{\text{in}}(\xi)$ can be represented as

$$f_{\text{out}}(t) = \int_{-\infty}^{+\infty} \hat{f}_{in}(\xi)\hat{h}(\xi)e^{2\pi i\xi t}d\xi = \int_{-\infty}^{+\infty} f_{\text{in}}(\tau)h(t-\tau)d\tau = (f_{in} * h)(t) \tag{4.1}$$

where $f_{\text{out}}(t)$ is the output time-domain signal, the unit of ξ is Hz, and $\hat{h}(\xi)$ is a frequency response function.

Following Eq. (4.1), the graph convolution operation on discrete graph node signal $\hat{h}(\lambda_k)$ can be defined as

$$f_{\text{out}}(i) = \sum_{k=1}^{n} \hat{f}_{in}(\lambda_k)\hat{h}(\lambda_k)v_k(i) \tag{4.2}$$

where $\hat{f}_{\text{in}}(\lambda_k)$ represents the strength of the graph signal at frequency λ_k, $v_k(\cdot)$ is the Fourier basis of the graph signal, i represents the i th element of $v_k(\cdot)$. In Eq. (4.2), the integral operation in Eq. (4.1) is replaced with the sum operation.

Let $\hat{f}_{in} = U^T f_{in}$, simplify Eq. (4.2) to matrix form as follows

$$\begin{aligned}
f_{\text{out}} &= \sum_{k=1}^{n} h(\lambda_k)\hat{f}_{\text{in}}(\lambda_k)\boldsymbol{v}_k = \begin{bmatrix} | & | & \dots & | \\ \boldsymbol{v}_1 & \boldsymbol{v}_2 & \dots & \boldsymbol{v}_n \\ | & | & \dots & | \end{bmatrix} \begin{bmatrix} h(\lambda_1)\hat{f}_{in}(\lambda_1) \\ h(\lambda_2)\hat{f}_{in}(\lambda_2) \\ \dots \\ h(\lambda_n)\hat{f}_{\text{in}}(\lambda_n) \end{bmatrix} \\
&= \begin{bmatrix} | & | & \dots & | \\ \boldsymbol{v}_1 & \boldsymbol{v}_2 & \dots & \boldsymbol{v}_n \\ | & | & \dots & | \end{bmatrix} \begin{bmatrix} h(\lambda_1) & \dots & 0 \\ \vdots & \ddots & \vdots \\ 0 & \dots & h(\lambda_n) \end{bmatrix} \begin{bmatrix} - & \boldsymbol{v}_1^T & - \\ - & \boldsymbol{v}_2^T & - \\ - & \dots & - \\ - & \boldsymbol{v}_n^T & - \end{bmatrix} f_{in} \\
&= \boldsymbol{U} \begin{bmatrix} h(\lambda_1) & \dots & 0 \\ \vdots & \ddots & \vdots \\ 0 & \dots & h(\lambda_n) \end{bmatrix} \boldsymbol{U}^T f_{\text{in}} = \boldsymbol{U}\boldsymbol{\Lambda}_h\boldsymbol{U}^T f_{in} = \mathbf{H} f_{\text{in}}
\end{aligned} \tag{4.3}$$

Accordingly, the graph filter can be defined as

$$\boldsymbol{H} = \boldsymbol{U}\boldsymbol{\Lambda}_{\text{h}}\boldsymbol{U}^{\text{T}} \in \mathbb{R}^{\text{n}\times\text{n}}, \boldsymbol{H} : \mathbb{R}^{\text{n}} \to \mathbb{R}^{\text{n}} \tag{4.4}$$

where $\boldsymbol{\Lambda}_{\text{h}}$ is the frequency response matrix of the graph filter.

4.2.3 Contrastive Learning

Contrastive learning learns deep semantic and feature information by comparing the similarities and differences between different samples, in which the input data is divided into different categories or groups (positive and negative sample pairs),

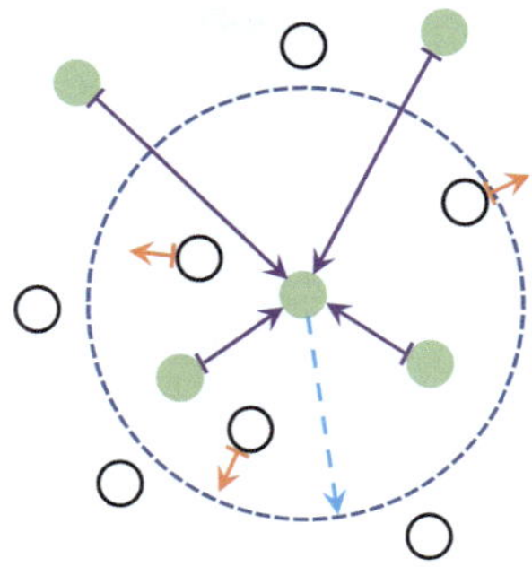

Fig. 4.1 The conceptual interpretation of contrastive learning (hollow nodes represent negative samples, while the solid nodes represent positive samples)

thus features are extracted and samples are classified, the conceptual interpretation is shown in Fig. 4.1.

Given a sample x, the core of contrastive learning is to learn a mapping function f satisfying the following condition

$$s\left(f(x), f\left(x^{+}\right)\right) >> s\left(f(x), f\left(x^{-}\right)\right) \tag{4.5}$$

where x^{+} and x^{-} are a positive sample similar to x and a negative sample dissimilar to x, respectively. $s(\cdot)$ is a function used to measure the similarity between samples.

4.3 Proposed Method

4.3.1 Problem Definition and Overview of SLCGC

The SLCGC framework integrates four core components: homogeneous region generation, low-pass spectral preservation, graph-based contrastive feature learning, and fused representation clustering. Figure 4.2 illustrates the end-to-end architecture, where each module synergistically interacts to optimize hyperspectral image (HSI) analysis. Below, we detail these components:

- **Homogeneous Region Generation**: A superpixel-based segmentation technique is employed to convert HSI data from pixel-level to region-level representations. This process retains local spatial-spectral coherence while significantly reducing computational complexity by minimizing node redundancy.
- **Low-pass Graph Denoising**: The superpixel-derived graph serves as input to a spectral preservation mechanism. To attenuate high-frequency noise and emphasize low-frequency structural patterns, neighborhood-based information propagation is implemented using adaptive graph filters, ensuring robust feature retention for subsequent clustering.

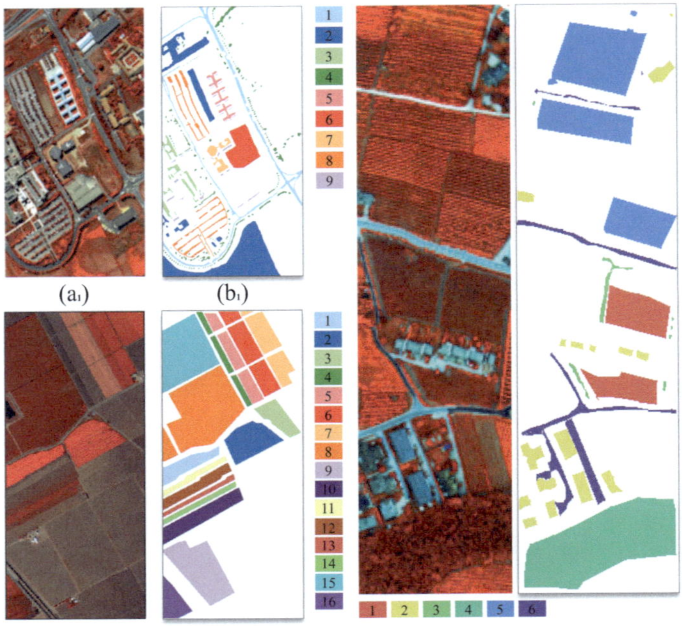

Fig. 4.2 Three dataset details. ($\mathbf{a}_1$), ($\mathbf{a}_2$), and ($\mathbf{a}_3$) are the false-color maps of PU, Salinas, and Trento datasets. ($\mathbf{b}_1$), ($\mathbf{b}_2$), and ($\mathbf{b}_3$) are the ground-truth maps. ($\mathbf{c}_1$), ($\mathbf{c}_2$), and ($\mathbf{c}_3$) are corresponding reference colors and containing pixels

- **Graph Structural Contrastive Learning**: Dual Siamese encoders with distinct parameters process the denoised graph features. Each branch incorporates dual MLP architectures to refine spectral-spatial attributes, while Gaussian noise perturbations generate divergent augmented views, enhancing feature diversity for discriminative learning.
- **Feature Fusion and Clustering**: A linear fusion strategy combines contrastive representations from both views. A cross-view consistency loss function is introduced to align structural semantics across embeddings, refining feature discriminability. Finally, latent features are partitioned via K-means to produce cluster assignments.

The SLCGC framework unifies these modules into a cohesive pipeline, enabling iterative refinement through inter-module feedback while maintaining computational efficiency for HSI applications.

4.3.2 Homogeneous Region Generation

HSI contains numerous pixels, which is computationally intensive if we take each pixel as input for the SLCGC. To solve this problem, superpixel segmentation is currently the most mainstream method. Thus, a superpixel segmentation method is proposed to generate homogeneous regions. Specifically, a linear discriminant analysis (LDA) [35] is first adopted to reduce the dimension of HSI for subsequent processing. Then, the simple linear iterative cluster (SLIC) [36] method is applied to divide the entire HSI into many spatially connected superpixels. Given an HSI $\boldsymbol{I} \in \mathbb{R}^{h \times w \times b}$, where h, w, and b represent the height, width, and number of bands of the HSI, respectively, we can transform HSI into an undirected graph $\mathcal{G} = \{\boldsymbol{X}, \boldsymbol{A}\}$ by treating each superpixel as a graph node and establishing nearest neighbor relationships between superpixels, where $N \ll h \times w$. Furthermore, the $\boldsymbol{X}$ is calculated as the average spectral features of the pixels contained in that superpixel. The $\boldsymbol{A} \in \mathbb{R}^{N \times N}$ is presented as

$$\boldsymbol{A}_{i,j} = \begin{cases} 1, & \text{if } S_i \text{ is adjacent to } S_j \\ 0, & \text{otherwise} \end{cases} \tag{4.6}$$

where $S_i = \{x_1^i, x_2^i, \ldots, x_{n_i}^i\}$ is the i th superpixel, n_i is the number of pixels contained in S_i.

To explore the connection between pixel and superpixel, an image backprojection operations are developed to transform data features from pixel to superpixel. Let $\boldsymbol{Q} \in \mathbb{R}^{hw \times N}$ is the correlation matrix introduced by SLIC, which is defined as

$$\boldsymbol{Q}_{i,j} = \begin{cases} 1, & \text{if } x_i \in S_i \\ 0, & \text{otherwise} \end{cases} \tag{4.7}$$

Graph projection can encode the original pixel level HSI into superpixel level graph node features through matrix multiplication, which can be represented as

$$\boldsymbol{V} = \text{Projection}(\boldsymbol{X}; \boldsymbol{Q}) = \hat{\boldsymbol{Q}}^T \text{Flatten}\,(\boldsymbol{X}) \tag{4.8}$$

where $\hat{\boldsymbol{Q}}$ is $\boldsymbol{Q}$ normalized by column, i.e., $\hat{Q}_{i,j} = Q_{i,j} / \sum_m Q_{m,j}$. Flatten$(\cdot)$ represents flattening HSI according to spatial dimensions.

4.3.3 Low-Pass Graph Denoising

Recently, graph filters have demonstrated a significant impact on graph convolution performance. Inspired by this, a low-pass graph denoising mechanism is designed to filter out noise interference in the graph structure and obtain a smoothed structure graph, with which we can efficiently filter out high-frequency noise in graph nodes.

Theorem 1 *The smoothness of graph signal* **X** *can be measured by Rayleigh quotient* [37], *namely*

$$R(\boldsymbol{L},\boldsymbol{X})=\frac{\boldsymbol{X}^{\top}\boldsymbol{L}\boldsymbol{X}}{\boldsymbol{X}^{\top}\boldsymbol{X}}=\frac{\sum_{(\boldsymbol{x}_i,\boldsymbol{x}_j)\in\mathcal{E}}\left(\boldsymbol{x}_i-\boldsymbol{x}_j\right)^2}{\sum_{i\in\mathcal{V}}\boldsymbol{x}_i^2} \tag{4.9}$$

Equation (4.9) can measure the similarity of node features between the two nodes in the graph, meaning that a smoother signal has a smaller Rayleigh quotient.

Theorem 2 *We can obtain a smoother signal by filtering high-frequency-basis signals, while preserving low-frequency-basis signals.*

According to Eq. (4.9), we can convert Theorem 2 to the following situation, for any node signal **X** and its filtered $\tilde{X}=\mathbf{HX}$ (frequency response function p(λ) of **H** is nonnegative and nonincreasing for all λ_i), always satisfy

$$R\big(\tilde{\boldsymbol{X}},\boldsymbol{X}\big)\le R(\boldsymbol{L},\boldsymbol{X}) \tag{4.10}$$

that is

$$\frac{\sum_{i=1}^{n}b_i\lambda_i}{\sum_{i=1}^{n}b_i}\le\frac{\sum_{c=1}^{n}c_i\lambda_i}{\sum_{c=1}^{n}c_i} \tag{4.11}$$

where b_i and c_i are the coefficient of eigenvector
λ_i. The induction is adopted, that is

$$\begin{aligned}R_b^i&=\frac{\sum_{i=1}^{n}b_i\lambda_i}{\sum_{i=1}^{n}b_i}\\ R_c^i&=\frac{\sum_{i=1}^{n}c_i\lambda_i}{\sum_{i=1}^{n}c_i}\end{aligned} \tag{4.12}$$

If, $\frac{c_1}{b_1}\le\cdots\le\frac{c_n}{b_n}$ and $\lambda_1\le\cdots\lambda_n$, hence $R_b^2\le R_c^2$. If $R_b^{l-1}\le R_c^{l-1}$ and $n=l-1$, the R_b^l can expressed as

$$\begin{aligned}\frac{\sum_{i=1}^{l}b_i\lambda_i}{\sum_{i=1}^{l}b_i}&=\frac{\sum_{i=1}^{l-1}b_i\lambda_i+b_l\lambda_l}{\sum_{i=1}^{l-1}b_i+b_l}\\ &=\frac{\left(\sum_{i=1}^{l-1}b_i\right)\lambda_b^{(l-1)}+b_l\lambda_l}{\sum_{i=1}^{l-1}b_i+b_l}\\ &\le\frac{\left(\sum_{i=1}^{l-1}b_i\right)\lambda_c^{(l-1)}+b\lambda_l}{\sum_{i=1}^{l-1}b_i+b_l}\end{aligned} \tag{4.13}$$

Since, $R_b^{l-1} \leq R_c^{l-1}$, and $\frac{\sum_{i=1}^{l-1} c_i}{\sum_{i=1}^{l-1} b_i} \leq \frac{c_l}{b_l}$, namely

$$\begin{aligned} \frac{\left(\sum_{i=1}^{l-1} b_i\right)\lambda_c^{(l-1)} + b\lambda_l}{\sum_{i=1}^{l-1} b_i + b_l} &\leq \frac{\left(\sum_{i=1}^{l-1} c_i\right)\lambda_c^{(l-1)} + c\lambda_l}{\sum_{i=1}^{l-1} c_i + c_l} \\ &= \frac{\sum_{i=1}^{l} c_i\lambda_i}{\sum_{i=1}^{l} c_i} \end{aligned} \tag{4.14}$$

Therefore, the Theorem 2 is proofed for all n.

Specifically, we can express the frequency response function as

$$p(\lambda_i) = 1 - k\lambda_i \tag{4.15}$$

where λ_i is the ith eigenvalues. Thus, a graph Laplacian filter in our chapter is introduced, namely

$$\boldsymbol{H} = \boldsymbol{U}p(\boldsymbol{\Lambda}_h)\boldsymbol{U}^T = \boldsymbol{U}(\boldsymbol{I} - k\boldsymbol{\Lambda}_h)\boldsymbol{U}^T = \boldsymbol{I} - k\tilde{\boldsymbol{L}} \tag{4.16}$$

where k is the coefficient parameter, $\tilde{\boldsymbol{L}}$ is the symmetric normalized graph Laplacian matrix. Afterward, t-layer graph Laplacian filters are stacked up, namely

$$\begin{aligned} X_t &= \left(\prod_{i=1} H\right)X \\ &= H^t X \end{aligned} \tag{4.17}$$

where $\boldsymbol{X}$ and $\boldsymbol{X}_t$ is original node feature and the smoothed node feature, respectively; $\boldsymbol{H}^t$ is t-layer stacked graph Laplacian filters, with which the low-pass spectral features can be preserved. Thus, the clustering performance is improved.

4.3.4 Graph Structural Contrastive Learning

To keep the structural consistency of the graph and reduce the computational complexity of the proposed method, a graph structural contrastive learning is proposed. Different from all previous methods, we don't use a graph convolutional neural network (GNN) to encode smoothed graph signals. Specifically, the smoothed node feature $\boldsymbol{X}_t$ is first encoded with two parameter un-shared MLP encoders. Subsequently, the ℓ^2-norm is applied to normalize the learned node features, which can be expressed as

$$\begin{aligned} \mathbf{Z}^{l_1} &= \text{MLP}_1(\mathbf{X}_t), \mathbf{Z}^{l_1} = \frac{\mathbf{Z}^{l_1}}{\mathbf{Z}_2^{l_1}} \\ \mathbf{Z}^{l_2} &= \text{MLP}_2(\mathbf{X}_t), \mathbf{Z}^{l_2} = \frac{\mathbf{Z}^{l_2}}{\mathbf{Z}_2^{l_2}} \end{aligned} \tag{4.18}$$

where $\mathbf{Z}^{l_1}$ and $\mathbf{Z}^{l_2}$ are two augmented views, l_1 and l_2 denote branch 1 and branch 2 of the contrastive learning. In our network, branch 1 and branch 2 do not share parameter, thus different semantic information would be contained during training.

The key to contrastive learning lies in how to construct positive and negative sample pairs reasonably and efficiently and maximize the semantic information covered by positive and negative sample pairs. Therefore, the random Gaussian noise.

$\mathbf{N} \in \mathbb{R}^{N \times d}$ is injected $\mathbf{Z}^{l_1}$ to keep to branch different as

$$\mathbf{Z}^{l_1} = \mathbf{Z}^{l_1} + \mathbf{N} \tag{4.19}$$

where $\mathbf{N}$ follows the distribution of $\mathcal{N}(0, \sigma)$. By leveraging Eq. (4.19), we generate two augmented representations while simultaneously improving the algorithm's robustness to noise interference.

4.3.5 Feature Fusion and Clustering

The contrastive node embedding features are learned in Sect. 4.3.4. Afterward, the two augmented views are fused with a linear manner, the resultant clustering-oriented node features $\mathbf{Z} \in \mathbb{R}^{N \times d}$ can be calculated as

$$\mathbf{Z} = \frac{1}{2}(\mathbf{Z}^{l_1} + \mathbf{Z}^{l_2}) \tag{4.20}$$

In our SLCGC, we can get the finally clustering results by performing K-means.

To enhance the structural consistency of the network and effectively train the network, a novel cross-view contrastive loss is designed. Specifically, a similarity matrix $\mathbf{S} \in \mathbb{R}^{N \times N}$ is calculated to evaluated the similarity between $\mathbf{Z}^{l_1}$ and $\mathbf{Z}^{l_2}$, namely

$$\mathbf{S}_{ij} = \mathbf{Z}_i^{l_1} \cdot \left(\mathbf{Z}_j^{l_2}\right)^{\mathrm{T}}, \forall i, j \in [1, N] \tag{4.21}$$

where $\mathbf{S}_{ij}$ measure the similarity between ith node feature in $\mathbf{Z}^{l_1}$ and jth node feature in $\mathbf{Z}^{l_2}$, which has the same meaning as the adjacency matrix in graph. Inspired by this, the cross-view contrastive loss can be constructed by minimizing the differences between $\mathbf{S}$ and self-looped adjacency matrix $\hat{\mathbf{A}} = \mathbf{I} + \mathbf{A} \in \mathbb{R}^{N \times N}$, namely

$$L = \frac{1}{N^2} \sum (S - \hat{\mathbf{A}})^2$$

$$= \frac{1}{N^2}\left(\sum_i \sum_j 1_{ij}^1 (\boldsymbol{S}_{ij} - 1)^2 + \sum_i \sum_j 1_{ij}^0 \boldsymbol{S}_{ij}^2\right) \tag{4.22}$$

where 1_{ij}^1 and 1_{ij}^0 denote $\hat{\boldsymbol{A}}_{ij} = 1$ and $\hat{\boldsymbol{A}}_{ij} = 0$. From Eq. (4.22), we can observe that, cross-view neighbors' nodes are considered as the positive samples, while the other non-neighbor nodes are regarded as negative samples. In our SLCGC, the Adam optimize [38] is introduced to minimize $\mathcal{L}$ during training. The learning process is detailed in Algorithm 1.

Algorithm 1: SLCGC for hyperspectral images

1: **Input**: The input HSI; Initial centroids (Cluster) number m; Iterations number T; Graph Laplacian filter layer t; Standard deviation of Gaussian noise σ
Output: Clustering results $\boldsymbol{Q}$

2: Initialization: $t = 2$; $\sigma = 0.01$;

3: Generate the homogeneous region and construct the superpixel-based graph by Eq. (4.6)-(4.8);

4: Apply t-layers low-pass graph filters on $\boldsymbol{X}$ to obtain the smoothed node feature $\boldsymbol{X}_t$ by Eq. (4.17);

5: **For** $t = 1$ to T do

6: The $\boldsymbol{X}_t$ is encoded by introducing graph structural contrastive learning, and then normalized by Eq. (4.18);

7: The random Gaussian noise is injected to perturb node embeddings by Eq. (4.19);

8: The similarity matrix $\boldsymbol{S}$ is calculated by Eq. (4.21);

9: The cross-view contrastive loss $\mathcal{L}$ is calculated by Eq. (4.22);

10: The clustering-oriented node features **Z** is obtained by Eq. (4.20);

11: The weight matrices are updated by minimizing $\mathcal{L}$ with Adam optimizer.

12: **End**

13: The clustering results $\boldsymbol{Q}$ is obtained by applying K-means on **Z**.

4.3.6 Computational Complexity Analysis

Let N be the graph node number, d be the spectral dimension of HSI, c be the cluster number, d_i is the dimensional of two MLPs. The computational complexity of low-pass graph denoising mechanism is $\mathcal{O}(Nd^2)$. For graph structural contrastive learning, the computational complexity is $\mathcal{O}(2Ndd_1 + 2Nd_1d_2)$. If SLCGC iterates T times during training, the overall computational complexity is

$\mathcal{O}\left[\left(Nd^2\right) + 2Nd_1(d + d_2)T\right]$. From the above derivation, it verifies that our proposed network contains high computational efficiency.

4.4 Experiments

This section presents a systematic evaluation of the SLCGC framework's efficacy through rigorous empirical investigations. The assessment protocol encompasses the following phases: (1) Dataset and Configuration Overview: Three benchmark HSI datasets and methodological configurations are detailed (Sects. 4.4.1–4.4.2); (2) Comparative Performance Benchmarking: Quantitative metrics and visual assessments are benchmarked against multiple leading-edge algorithms to validate clustering superiority (Sect. 4.4.3); (3) Ablation Analysis: Component-specific ablation studies verify the architectural rationality of SLCGC (Sect. 4.4.4); (4) Hyperparameter Sensitivity: The impact of parameter configurations on model stability is explored (Sect. 4.4.5); (5) Spatial-Semantic Visualization: Cluster characterization outcomes are presented to interpret spatial coherence (Sect. 4.4.6); (6) Computational Efficiency: Runtime and resource demands across examined deep clustering frameworks are benchmarked (Sect. 4.4.7).

4.4.1 Benchmark Datasets

In our experiments, three well-known HSI datasets were adopted, including the Salinas dataset, the Pavia University (PU) dataset, and the Trento dataset, which are briefly summarized in Fig. 4.2.

4.4.2 Experiment Setup

For benchmarking purposes, a suite of contemporary clustering models was selected, encompassing conventional approaches (k-means [20], Fuzzy c-means [21], spectral clustering [39]), subspace-based techniques (SSSC [40], NCSC [41]), deep learning frameworks (SDCN [42], NCSC), and graph autoencoder architectures (EGAE [43], AdaGAE [44]). Within the SLCGC framework, five critical hyperparameters required initialization: iteration cycles (T), learning rate (L), Laplacian filter layers (t), Gaussian noise intensity (σ), and MLP embedding dimensions (d_i). Optimal configurations, detailed in Table 4.2, are further examined in Sect. 4.4.5.

All trials were executed on an NVIDIA Titan RTX GPU utilizing PyTorch to ensure computational consistency. To mitigate stochastic variability, each method underwent ten independent runs with randomized training samples.

Table 4.2 Preset optimal parameters in SLCGC

Dataset	T	L	t	σ	d_i
Salinas	400	1e−3	2	0.01	500
PU	400	1e−3	2	0.01	500
Trento	400	1e−3	2	0.01	500

.Performance evaluation employed six established metrics: Overall Accuracy (OA), Per-Class Accuracy (PA), Kappa coefficient (κ), Normalized Mutual Information (NMI), Adjusted Rand Index (ARI), and Purity. Additionally, classification maps were generated to facilitate visual comparisons of clustering outcomes across models.

4.4.3 Comparative Experimental Results and Analysis

Building on the experimental configurations outlined in Sect. 4.4.5, clustering analyses were conducted across the Salinas, PU, and Trento datasets. Tabulated results (Tables 4.3, 4.4 and 4.5) summarize the mean and standard deviation values for six metrics: PA, OA, κ, NMI, ARI, and Purity, with top performances highlighted in bold and runner-up entries underlined.

Salinas Dataset Evaluation: Initial evaluations focus on the Salinas dataset to validate SLCGC's efficacy. Metric-driven and visual outcomes are cataloged in Table 4.3 and Fig. 4.3. Quantitative results reveal SLCGC's superiority, achieving 85.48% (OA), 83.77% (κ), 88.81% (ARI), and 86.01% (Purity)—surpassing the second-best performers (NCSC and EGAE) by margins of 6.67%, 7.75%, 16.98%, and 2.44%, respectively. While NCSC, EGAE, and AdaGAE exhibit moderate noise resilience and adaptability to class distribution skews, conventional techniques like FCM and SSSC underperform due to their lack of HSI-specific design. Traditional methods (k-means, FCM, SC) yield subpar results (e.g., OAs of 67.99%, 56.73%, 52.68%), attributed to limited high-level feature extraction. SDCN's integration of graph structures fails to exploit spectral-pixel relationships adequately. SLCGC's low-pass denoising mechanism mitigates high-frequency noise, corroborated by Fig. 4.3, where its outputs display fewer misclassifications (e.g., reduced "salt-and-pepper" artifacts in Weed 1/2 and Fallow regions) compared to error-prone maps from competitors like NCSC in Grapes untrained zones.

PU Dataset Analysis: The PU dataset, characterized by compact terrain distribution, posed heightened clustering challenges. As Table 4.4 and Fig. 4.5 illustrate, SLCGC attained leading scores (68.23% (OA), 58.70% (κ), 63.92% (NMI), 52.32% (ARI), 75.36% (Purity)), outperforming the second-best methods by 13.04%, 6.24%, 8.63%, 13.63%, and 5.24%, respectively. Notably, k-means demonstrated moderate efficacy despite deep frameworks (NCSC, SDCN) struggling with limited feature

Table 4.3 Quantitative experimental classification results on salinas, the best performances and the second-best performances are marked in bold and underline

No	k-means	SC	FCM	SSSC	NCSC	SDCN	EGAE	AdaGAE	SLCGC
1	0.9985	0.5726	0.4179	0.0416	0.0000	0.0000	**1.0000**	0.0000	**1.0000**
2	0.5698	0.4982	0.5524	0.9875	**1.0000**	**1.0000**	**1.0000**	0.9997	**1.0000**
3	0.9741	0.5976	0.8501	0.0154	0.6822	0.3426	**1.0000**	**1.0000**	**1.0000**
4	**0.9865**	0.0133	0.0000	0.8131	0.0000	0.0000	0.0000	0.0000	0.0000
5	0.7856	0.6810	0.5540	0.8723	**0.9988**	0.9816	0.0000	0.9572	0.9922
6	0.9952	0.9722	**0.9990**	0.9358	0.9941	0.9530	0.9886	0.9900	0.9914
7	0.4810	0.0000	0.0000	0.5412	**1.0000**	0.0000	0.9983	0.9999	0.9916
8	0.7309	0.7291	0.7772	0.4226	0.8026	0.7633	0.5131	0.5631	**0.9183**
9	0.9750	0.5493	0.6969	0.5638	0.9076	0.8643	0.8326	0.9832	**0.9985**
10	0.6169	0.2683	0.5507	0.1143	0.9900	0.5519	0.8962	0.9000	**0.9323**
11	0.3370	0.0000	0.0000	0.6915	**0.9531**	0.0000	0.0000	0.8702	0.8970
12	0.0273	0.0000	0.0047	0.4857	0.0000	0.2287	**1.0000**	0.4926	0.8858
13	0.3548	0.7597	**0.8134**	0.0000	0.0000	0.0690	0.0000	0.0000	0.0000
14	0.5584	0.6815	0.6512	0.1826	0.0000	**0.7632**	0.0000	0.0000	0.0000
15	0.4994	0.3601	0.4279	0.4682	0.8563	0.0980	**0.9692**	0.9436	0.5989
16	0.0000	0.7932	0.8321	0.9265	**1.0000**	0.0000	**1.0000**	0.9575	**1.0000**
OA (%)	0.6799	0.5268	0.5673	0.5243	0.7881	0.5382	0.7361	0.7683	**0.8548**
Kappa	0.6572	0.4839	0.5431	0.5069	0.7602	0.4793	0.7106	0.7382	**0.8377**
NMI	0.7356	0.6123	0.6859	0.6423	0.8514	0.6589	**0.8769**	0.8251	0.7660
ARI	0.5466	0.4297	0.4693	0.4676	0.7068	0.4831	0.7183	0.6532	**0.8881**
Purity	0.7132	0.6410	0.7016	0.6819	0.7893	0.5765	0.8357	0.8002	**0.8601**

extraction in spatially constrained contexts. SLCGC's dual MLP architecture leverages smoothed structural and global–local semantic correlations, yielding superior accuracy. Visualizations confirm its alignment with ground-truth labels and reduced misclassification rates.

Trento Dataset Assessment: On the Trento dataset (Table 4.5, Fig. 4.4), SLCGC demonstrates robust performance, exceeding second-place benchmarks by 13.36% (OA), 17.05% (κ), 11.26% (NMI), 18.31% (ARI), and 2.59% (Purity). AdaGAE and NCSC delivered competitive results (e.g., NCSC: 74.89% (OA), 67.90% (κ)) through adaptive graph-based semantic extraction and nonlinear spatial mapping. However, SLCGC's noise-augmented dual-view contrastive framework and structural consistency optimization enhance feature discriminability and noise immunity. Figure 4.5 validates its visual dominance, with clustering maps closely mirroring ground-truth distributions.

Table 4.4 Quantitative experimental classification results on PU, the best performances and the second-best performances are marked in bold and underline

No	k-means	SC	FCM	SSSC	NCSC	SDCN	EGAE	AdaGAE	SLCGC
1	0.8234	0.7291	0.5732	0.2971	0.4238	0.6234	0.3029	<u>0.8521</u>	**0.8887**
2	0.3581	0.2196	0.3265	0.5867	<u>0.5933</u>	0.3803	0.5012	0.5329	**0.7488**
3	0.2167	0.0000	0.0024	0.3571	0.6902	0.1687	**0.9900**	<u>0.7194</u>	0.5000
4	0.5943	0.5791	0.5367	0.2612	0.0270	0.4025	0.2744	<u>0.7237</u>	**0.7507**
5	0.6620	0.6280	0.7124	0.0000	0.9735	0.6610	**1.0000**	0.0000	<u>0.9918</u>
6	0.4255	0.0000	0.3529	0.3128	<u>0.9711</u>	0.3328	**1.0000**	0.4932	0.2551
7	0.0000	<u>0.9213</u>	**0.9578**	0.0000	0.3382	0.3622	0.0000	0.0000	0.0000
8	**0.9608**	0.8462	0.8730	0.5182	0.4027	0.4729	0.6258	0.2320	<u>0.9503</u>
9	**0.9990**	0.0000	0.0000	0.8848	0.0000	0.3702	0.0000	0.4538	<u>0.9620</u>
OA (%)	0.5237	0.4192	0.4359	0.4032	<u>0.5519</u>	0.4207	0.5328	0.5436	**0.6823**
Kappa	<u>0.5246</u>	0.3968	0.4327	0.4187	0.4570	0.3185	0.4536	0.4139	**0.5870**
NMI	<u>0.5529</u>	0.4830	0.5126	0.4889	0.4392	0.4362	0.5372	0.4628	**0.6392**
ARI	0.3188	0.2372	0.2632	0.2537	<u>0.3869</u>	0.2399	0.3780	0.3271	**0.5232**
Purity	<u>0.7012</u>	0.6259	0.6785	0.6440	0.6638	0.6400	0.7126	0.6689	**0.7536**

Table. 4.5 Quantitative experimental classification results on Trento, the best performances and the second-best performances are marked in bold and underline

No	k-means	SC	FCM	SSSC	NCSC	SDCN	EGAE	AdaGAE	SLCGC
1	0.0000	0.0000	0.0000	<u>0.8235</u>	**1.0000**	0.2218	0.6522	**1.0000**	**1.0000**
2	0.0189	0.0000	0.0000	0.0000	0.0793	**0.7826**	<u>0.6029</u>	0.4826	0.2621
3	0.0000	0.0019	0.0000	0.0000	0.0000	<u>0.0359</u>	**0.0931**	0.0000	0.0000
4	0.7200	0.6265	0.6826	0.8792	**1.0000**	0.6237	0.9540	0.9622	<u>0.9954</u>
5	0.6182	0.1987	0.2007	0.3987	0.6437	<u>0.7452</u>	0.5196	0.6158	**0.9990**
6	0.0199	0.1280	0.0329	0.7653	**0.8206**	0.5930	0.3412	<u>0.8029</u>	0.7927
OA (%)	0.6301	0.4872	0.5132	0.6842	0.7489	0.6200	0.6487	<u>0.7562</u>	**0.8898**
Kappa	0.6026	0.4708	0.4917	0.6196	0.6790	0.5132	0.5380	<u>0.6810</u>	**0.8515**
NMI	0.4928	0.4235	0.4654	0.6726	<u>0.7312</u>	0.4860	0.6801	0.7250	**0.8438**
ARI	0.3457	0.2794	0.2802	0.6501	<u>0.7111</u>	0.4362	0.6624	0.6455	**0.8942**
Purity	0.6499	0.5129	0.6708	0.7832	<u>0.8652</u>	0.7050	0.8273	0.7726	**0.8911**

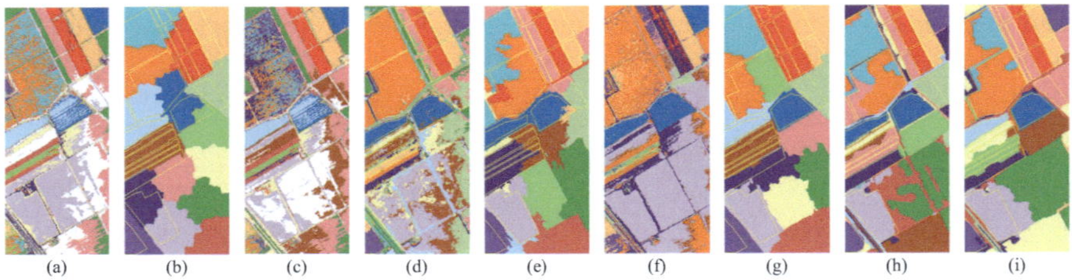

Fig. 4.3 Clustering maps of comparison methods on Salinas dataset. **a** k-means (OA = 67.99%); **b** SC (OA = 52.68%); **c** FCM (OA = 56.73%); **d** SSSC (OA = 52.43%); **e** NCSC (OA = 78.81%); **f** SDCN (OA = 53.82%); **g** EGAE (OA = 73.61%); **h** AdaGAE (OA = 76.83%); **i** SLCGC (OA = 85.48)

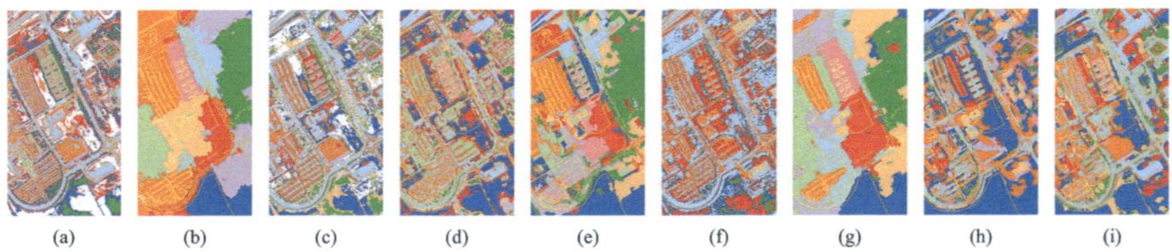

Fig. 4.4 Clustering maps of comparison methods on PU dataset. **a** k means (OA = 52.37%); **b** SC (OA = 41.92%); **c** FCM (OA = 43.59%); **d** SSSC(OA = 40.32%); **e** NCSC (OA = 55.19%); **f** SDCN (OA = 42.07%); **g** EGAE (OA = 53.28%); **h** AdaGAE (OA = 54.36%); **i** SLCGC (OA = 68.23)

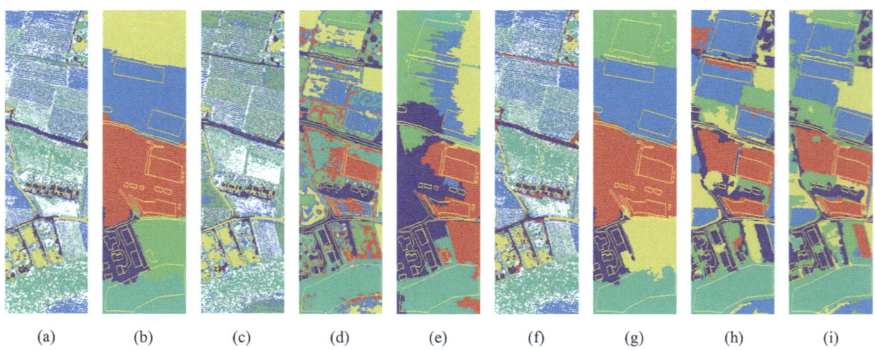

Fig. 4.5 Clustering maps of comparison methods on Trento dataset. **a** k-means (OA=63.01%); **b** SC (OA = 48.72%); **c** FCM (OA = 51.32%); **d** SSSC (OA = 68.42%); **e** NCSC (OA = 74.89%); **f** SDCN (OA = 62.00%); **g** EGAE (OA = 64.87%); **h** AdaGAE (OA = 75.62%); **i** SLCGC (OA = 88.98)

4.4.4 Ablation Studies

The SLCGC framework comprises four integral components: homogeneous region generation (GHR), low-pass graph denoising (LGD), graph structural contrastive

Table 4.6 Ablation study. ✓: Included block. ✗: Unincluded block

Name		SLCGC -v_1	SLCGC -v_2	SLCGC -v_3	SLCGC -v_4	SLCGC
Module	GHR	✗	✓	✓	✓	✓
	LGD	✓	✗	✓	✓	✓
	GSCL	✓	✓	✗	✓	✓
	G	✓	✓	✓	✗	✓
Dataset	Salinas (%)	78.39	71.74	72.35	73.35	**85.48**
	PU (%)	59.26	62.60	61.97	60.19	**68.23**
	Trento (%)	80.42	71.59	73.21	78.92	**88.98**

learning (GSCL), and feature fusion with clustering. To evaluate their individual contributions, ablation studies were conducted by sequentially removing each module and analyzing performance degradation. Additionally, the integration of Gaussian noise (G) amplifies feature robustness. In this part, we will evaluate their contribution to the overall clustering performance and a set of ablation studies have been conducted. Thus, SLCGC-V_1: Excludes the homogeneous region generation module, SLCGC-V_2: Removes the low-pass graph denoising mechanism (LGD), SLCGC-V_3: Omits the graph structural contrastive learning block (GSCL), SLCGC-V4: Eliminates Gaussian noise injection. As shown in Table 4.6, we can observe that (1) All ablated variants exhibit reduced accuracy across metrics compared to the full SLCGC framework, underscoring the necessity of each module; (2) The magnitude of performance degradation differs among variants, indicating distinct roles for GHR, LGD, GSCL, and G in optimizing clustering efficacy; (3) Every component enhances accuracy, validating their collective importance in addressing spatial-spectral complexity and noise resilience. This analysis confirms that the methodological innovations in SLCGC—homogeneous region generation, spectral denoising, contrastive feature learning, and noise-augmented fusion—collectively drive its superior clustering performance.

4.4.5 Hyper-Parameter Study

The SLCGC framework requires initialization of five critical hyperparameters (i.e., T, L, t, σ, d_i), with optimal configurations detailed in Table 4.2. This section elucidates their selection rationale and evaluates model sensitivity to these parameters. A systematic grid search was executed, guided by Overall Accuracy (OA) as the primary metric.

The number of epochs T and learning rate L control the number of cycles of the algorithm and the step-size of parameter optimization, respectively. Therefore, we conducted the experiments to access the sensitivity of two paraments varying T from 200 to 600 and L from 0.1×10^{-3} to 10×10^{-3}. And, the other hyper-parameters are fixed as in Table 4.2. In the results Fig. 4.6, we note that (1) the OA is highest when

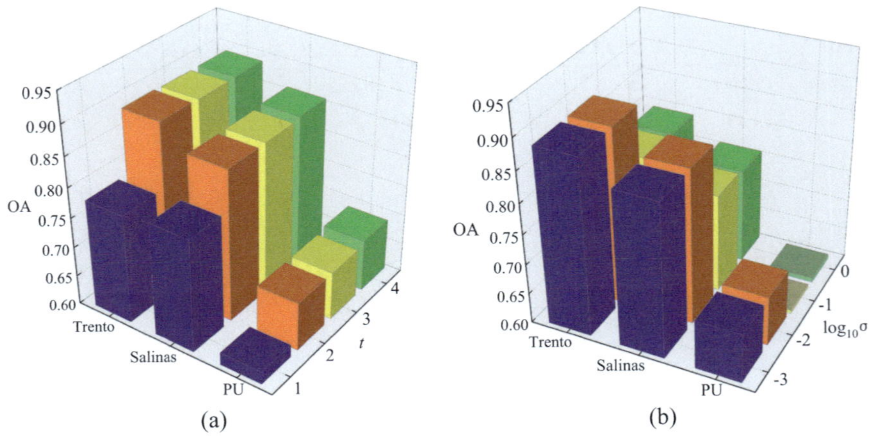

Fig. 4.6 Hyperparameter sensitivity analyses on three datasets. **a** graph Laplacian filter layer t. **b** standard deviation σ

T and L are 400 and 10^{-3}, respectively; (2) T and L are closely related, different T and L have a significant impact on clustering results; (3) a larger T and L can make the model more fully trained, but easy to lead to over-fitting. A smaller T and L may lead to insufficient optimization of the algorithm parameters. To ensure the training efficiency, 'while obtaining an optimistic clustering result, we preset T and L as 400 and 10^{-3}, respectively.

The number of graph Laplacian filter layer t is closely related to graph noise filtering. In this experiment, we investigate the impacts of different t for HSI clustering, and the results are shown in Fig. 4.6a. In general, larger t can filter more high-frequency noise in the graph, while accompanying greater computational complexity. Thus, the appropriate t is 2. The standard deviation of Gaussian noise σ is used to provide negative samples for contrastive learning. After that, we analyze the effect of the σ. From the results in Fig. 4.6b, we can observe that the clustering results decreases drastically as $\sigma > 0.1$, mainly because the node embedding semantic drift as too much noise injected. The results indicate that the optimistic value of σ is 0.1.

4.4.6 T-SNE Data Distributions Visualization

In this section, the t-distributed stochastic neighbor embedding (t-SNE) [43] method is employed to visualize the distribution of graph nodes in three datasets to validate the clustering performance of SLCGC. From Fig. 4.7a–c are the original distribution of original graph nodes, while (d–f) represent the distribution of graph node features after processing with SLCGC. By comparing and analyzing, the following conclusion can be drawn: (1) Post-processing (d–f) exhibits reduced inter-class variance versus

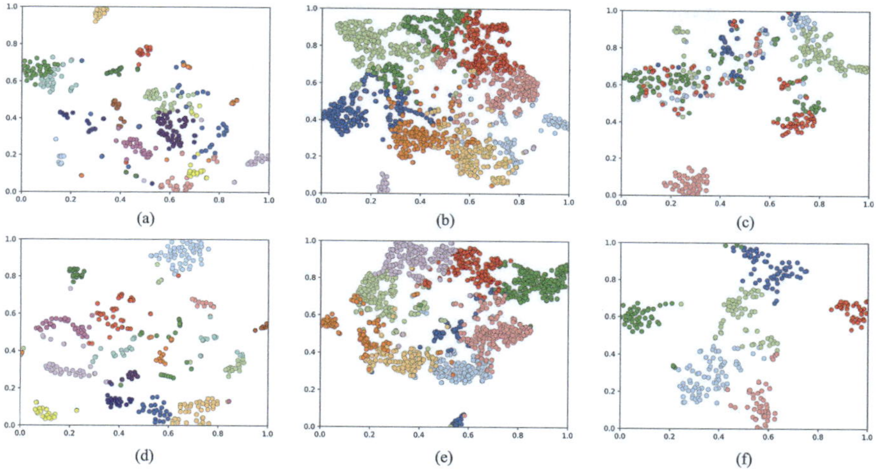

Fig. 4.7 Visualization of SLCGC using t-SNE on SA (**a**, **d**), PU (**b**, **e**), and Trento (**c**, **f**). **a**–**c** are original distributions of three datasets. **d**–**f** are distributions after clustering. Different color nodes within the maps denote different land covers

raw data (a–c), confirming enhanced cluster coherence; (2) Increased inter-class separation and intra-class compactness in (d–f) reflect refined structural organization; (3) Distinct landcover differentiation underscores SLCGC's efficacy in spatial-spectral disentanglement. Thus, graph nodes processed by SLCGC exhibit tighter intraclass compactness and more considerable inter-class distances. Furthermore, the clustering task mentioned in Eq. (4.6) is effectively implemented.

4.4.7 Complexity Comparison

Comparative analysis (Table 4.7) of training duration, inference speed, and FLOPs reveals SLCGC's superior efficiency. Its reduced complexity and resource demands validate practical viability, achieving high accuracy without computational overhead.

Table 4.7 Complexity comparison of deep learning methods(s)

Name	Salinas			PU			Trento		
	Train/s	Test/s	FLOPs	Train/s	Test/s	FLOPs	Train/s	Test/s	FLOPs
AdaGAE	144.8671	43.5324	130.02 M	1200.819	101.3368	1.29G	86.2017	13.7605	25.53 M
EAGE	199.946	4.8399	270.38 M	1763.686	39.8889	2.63G	186.1897	4.7581	57.09 M
NCSC	681.0274	15.6768	303.18G	1375.568	33.2784	596.49G	677.5501	19.3583	273.67G
SDCN	437.5881	0.6087	446.1G	274.8834	0.2034	339.56G	145.6749	0.3492	236.22G
SLCGC	44.4307	0.0010	44.1 M	160.0160	0.0010	31.4 M	43.8490	0.0009	13.08 M

4.5 Conclusion

This study introduces a computationally efficient self-supervised graph clustering framework (SLCGC) for hyperspectral imagery (HSI), leveraging low-pass contrastive mechanisms without convolutional layers. The methodology unfolds through four key phases: (1) Pixel-based data is transformed into region-based segments, preserving spatial-spectral coherence while minimizing graph complexity, (2) A graph-based module employs low-pass filters to attenuate high-frequency interference, enhancing robustness to noise, (3) Dual Siamese encoders with distinct parameters and a two-layer MLP architecture generate augmented representations, with Gaussian noise perturbations introducing negative samples for contrastive learning, (4) A linear fusion strategy combines augmented data, while a cross-view consistency loss strengthens structural alignment during training. Latent embeddings are subsequently clustered via K-means. Integrated into an end-to-end network, these components synergistically improve clustering accuracy, computational efficiency, and noise resilience, as evidenced by experimental validation.

Future Directions: Subsequent research will explore streamlined techniques for contrastive graph learning to reduce computational overhead. Additionally, reinforcement learning strategies may optimize HSI preprocessing, augmenting feature extraction capabilities for clustering tasks.

References

1. Ran R, Deng L-J, Zhang T-J, Chang J, Wu X, Tian Q (2024) KNLConv: kernel-space non-local convolution for hyperspectral image super-resolution. IEEE Trans Multimed 26:8836–8848
2. Hong D, Zhang B, Li X, Li Y, Li C, Yao J, Yokoya N, Li H, Ghamisi P, Jia X (2024) SpectralGPT: spectral remote sensing foundation model. IEEE Trans Pattern Anal Mach Intell 46:5227–5244
3. Zhang Y, Jiang G, Cai Z, Zhou Y (2024) Bipartite graph-based projected clustering with local region guidance for hyperspectral imagery. IEEE Trans Multimed 26:9551–9563
4. Ding Y, Zhao X, Zhang Z, Cai W, Yang N, Zhan Y (2021) Semi-supervised locality preserving dense graph neural network with ARMA filters and context-aware learning for hyperspectral image classification. IEEE Trans Geosci Remote Sens 60:1–12
5. Bai J, Shi W, Xiao Z, Ali TAA, Ye F, Jiao L (2023) Achieving better category separability for hyperspectral image classification: a spatial–spectral approach. IEEE Trans Neural Netw Learn Syst 35:9621–9635
6. Gao L, Hu H-M, Xue X, Hu H (2024) From appearance to inherence: a hyperspectral image dataset and benchmark of material classiffcation for surveillance. IEEE Trans Multimed 26:8569–8580
7. Li J, Bioucas-Dias JM, Plaza A (2012) Semisupervised hyperspectral image classification using soft sparse multinomial logistic regression. IEEE Geosci Remote Sens Lett 10(2):318–322
8. Ma L, Crawford MM, Tian J (2010) Local manifold learning-based k-nearest-neighbor for hyperspectral image classification. IEEE Trans Geosci Remote Sens 48(11):4099–4109
9. Tarabalka Y, Fauvel M, Chanussot J, Benediktsson JA (2010) SVM-and MRF-based method for accurate classification of hyperspectral images. IEEE Geosci Remote Sens Lett 7(4):736–740
10. Xia J, Ghamisi P, Yokoya N, Iwasaki A (2017) Random forest ensembles and extended multi-extinction profiles for hyperspectral image classification. IEEE Trans Geosci Remote Sens 56(1):202–216

11. Hu W, Huang YY, Wei L, Zhang F, Li HC (2015) Deep convolutional neural networks for hyperspectral image classification. J Sens
12. Yang A, Li M, Ding Y, Hong D, Lv Y, He Y (2023) GTFN: GCN and transformer fusion with spatial-spectral features for hyperspectral image classification. IEEE Trans Geosci Rem Sens
13. Liu Q, Peng J, Chen N, Sun W, Ning Y, Du Q (2023) Category-specific prototype self-refinement contrastive learning for few-shot hyperspectral image classification. IEEE Trans Geosci Remote Sens 61:1–16
14. Ding Y, Zhang Z, Zhao X, Cai W, Yang N, Hu H, Huang X, Cao Y, Cai W (2022) Unsupervised self-correlated learning smoothy enhanced locality preserving graph convolution embedding clustering for hyperspectral images. IEEE Trans Geosci Remote Sens 60:1–16
15. Zhang Y, Wang Y, Chen X, Jiang X, Zhou Y (2022) Spectral–spatial feature extraction with dual graph autoencoder for hyperspectral image clustering. IEEE Trans Circuits Syst Video Technol 32(12):8500–8511
16. Liu Q, Peng J, Zhang G, Sun W, Du Q (2023) Deep contrastive learning network for small-sample hyperspectral image classification. J Rem Sens 3:0025
17. Tu W, Zhou S, Liu X, Guo X, Cai Z, Zhu E, Cheng J (2021) Deep fusion clustering network. Proc AAAI Conf Artif Intell 35(11):9978–9987
18. Tu W, Guan R, Zhou S, Ma C, Peng X, Cai Z, Liu Z, Cheng J, Liu X (2024) Attribute-missing graph clustering network. Proc AAAI Conf Artif Intell 38(14):15392–15401
19. Zhongdong W, Xinbo G, Weixin X, Jianping Y (2005) Kernel method-based fuzzy clustering algorithm. J Syst Eng Electron 16(1):160–166
20. Kanungo T, Mount DM, Netanyahu NS, Piatko CD, Silverman R, Wu AY (2002) An efficient k-means clustering algorithm: analysis and implementation. IEEE Trans Pattern Anal Mach Intell 24(7):881–892
21. Yang T-n, Lee C-j, Yen S-j (2009) Fuzzy objective functions for robust pattern recognition. In: 2009 IEEE international conference on fuzzy systems, pp 2057–2062
22. Li Q, Liu W, Li L (2018) Affinity learning via a diffusion process for subspace clustering. Pattern Recogn 84:39–50
23. Liu Y, Yang X, Zhou S, Liu X, Wang S, Liang K, Tu W, Li L (2023) Simple contrastive graph clustering. IEEE Trans Neural Netw Learn Syst
24. Zhang H, Zhai H, Zhang L, Li P (2016) Spectral–spatial sparse subspace clustering for hyperspectral remote sensing images. IEEE Trans Geosci Remote Sens 54(6):3672–3684
25. Zhai H, Zhang H, Zhang L, Li P, Plaza A (2016) A new sparse subspace clustering algorithm for hyperspectral remote sensing imagery. IEEE Geosci Remote Sens Lett 14(1):43–47
26. Zhao Y, Li X (2023) Deep spectral clustering with regularized linear embedding for hyperspectral image clustering. IEEE Trans Geosci Rem Sens 61:1–11
27. Hu X, Li T, Zhou T, Peng Y (2021) Deep spatial-spectral subspace clustering for hyperspectral images based on contrastive learning. Rem Sens 13(21):4418
28. Cai Y, Zeng M, Cai Z, Liu X, Zhang Z (2021) Graph regularized residual subspace clustering network for hyperspectral image clustering. Inf Sci 578:85–101
29. Cai Y, Zhang Z, Cai Z, Liu X, Jiang X, Yan Q (2020) Graph convolutional subspace clustering: A robust subspace clustering framework for hyperspectral image. IEEE Trans Geosci Remote Sens 59(5):4191–4202
30. Wang Q, Miao Y, Chen M, Yuan Y (2022) Spatial-spectral clustering with anchor graph for hyperspectral image. IEEE Trans Geosci Remote Sens 60:1–13
31. Luo F, Zhang L, Du B, Zhang L (2020) Dimensionality reduction with enhanced hybrid-graph discriminant learning for hyperspectral image classification. IEEE Trans Geosci Remote Sens 58(8):5336–5353
32. Guan R, Li Z, Tu W, Wang J, Liu Y, Li X, Tang C, Feng R (2024) Contrastive multi-view subspace clustering of hyperspectral images based on graph convolutional networks. IEEE Trans Geosci Remote Sens 62:1–14
33. Ding Y, Zhang ZL, Zhao XF, Cai YM, Li SY, Deng B, Cai WW (2022) Self-supervised locality preserving low-pass graph convolutional embedding for large-scale hyperspectral image clustering. IEEE Trans Geosci Rem Sens 60

34. Guan R, Tu W, Li Z, Yu H, Hu D, Chen Y, Tang C, Yuan Q, Liu X (2024) Spatial-spectral graph contrastive clustering with hard sample mining for hyperspectral images. IEEE Trans Geosci Remote Sens 62:1–14
35. Izenman AJ (2013) Linear discriminant analysis. In: Modern multivariate statistical techniques. Springer, pp 237–280
36. Achanta R, Shaji A, Smith K, Lucchi A, Fua P, Süsstrunk S (2012) SLIC superpixels compared to state-of-the-art superpixel methods. IEEE Trans Pattern Anal Mach Intell 34(11):2274–2282
37. Horn RA, Johnson CR (2012) Matrix analysis. Cambridge University Press
38. Kingma DP, Ba J (2014) Adam: a method for stochastic optimization. arXiv preprint arXiv: 1412.6980
39. Ng A, Jordan M, Weiss Y (2001) On spectral clustering: analysis and an algorithm. In: Advances in neural information processing systems, vol 14
40. Peng X, Tang H, Zhang L, Yi Z, Xiao S (2015) A unified framework for representation-based subspace clustering of out-of-sample and large-scale data. IEEE Trans Neural Netw Learn Syst 27(12):2499–2512
41. Cai Y, Zhang Z, Ghamisi P, Ding Y, Liu X, Cai Z, Gloaguen R (2022) Superpixel contracted neighborhood contrastive subspace clustering network for hyperspectral images. IEEE Trans Geosci Remote Sens 60:1–13
42. Bo D, Wang X, Shi C, Zhu M, Lu E, Cui P, Structural deep clustering network, pp 1400–1410
43. Zhang H, Li P, Zhang R, Li X (2022) Embedding graph auto-encoder for graph clustering. IEEE Trans Neural Netw Learn Syst
44. Li X, Zhang H, Zhang R (2021) Adaptive graph auto-encoder for general data clustering. IEEE Trans Pattern Anal Mach Intell 44(12):9725–9732

Chapter 5
Self-Supervised Graph Convolutional with Locality Preserving Low-Pass Embedding for Large-Scale Hyperspectral Image Clustering

5.1 Introduction

Hyperspectral images (HSI) captured via remote sensing systems contain numerous consecutive narrow spectral bands, offering rich spatial-spectral data across the electromagnetic spectrum [1–3]. Given their distinct benefits, HSI has gained significant interest and found broad utilization in domains like military surveillance, urban planning, biochemical analysis, wildfire monitoring, and object identification [4–6].

Hyperspectral image classification (HSIC), a core technique for HSI analysis, seeks to categorize individual pixels into distinct land-cover types without prior labels. Recent advances in supervised and semi-supervised deep learning approaches for HSIC have demonstrated notable results [7, 8]. Yet, these techniques demand extensive annotated data for model training. Acquiring labeled HSI pixels remains highly laborious and time-intensive, posing a critical limitation for real-world HSIC deployment. Consequently, unsupervised clustering methods which group analogous pixels into land-cover categories without labeled references have grown in prominence. Unlike supervised counterparts, HSI clustering presents inherent challenges stemming from the lack of prior knowledge, significant spectral variations, and the high-dimensional nature of HSI data [9, 10].

In the past several decades, various clustering methods have been designed for HSI clustering [11, 12]. In the early stage, some traditional clustering algorithms developed for natural images have been applied to HSI clustering, such as k-means [13], spectral clustering (SC) [14], fuzzy c-means (FCM) [15], independent component analysis model (ICA) [16], FCM incorporating spatial-contextual information (FCM-S1) [17], etc. However, these algorithms only extract spectral information, the spatial information contained in HSI is ignored, which limits their performances. Thus, to fully utilize the spectral-spatial information of HSI and improve the clustering accuracy, some spectral-spatial HSI clustering methods [18–20] are designed, and better performances have been achieved than that of only spectral-based methods. Furthermore, to solve the high-dimensional problem of HSI, some sparse subspace

Y. Ding et al., *Graph Neural Network for Hyperspectral Image Clustering*, Intelligent Perception and Information Processing, https://doi.org/10.1007/978-981-96-7710-8_5

clustering (SSC) algorithms [21–23] have appeared, which can cluster the pixels in the low-dimensional subspace by learning the coefficient representation matrix and constructing the affinity matrix. In addition, Zhai et al. [24] integrated the total variation and collaborative subspace clustering (CSC) into a unified framework to present the spectral-spatial information of HSIs.

Regrettably, the methods mentioned above are shallow classifiers relying on hand-crafted features or raw feature spaces. They are unable to learn the high-level features of HSI and are not apt for effectively characterizing the extensive spectral variability and intricate internal structure of HSI datasets as stated in [25, 26]. Consequently, certain deep learning techniques have been employed to surmount this limitation. Given the successful implementation of deep-learning-based clustering in natural image clustering, several deep learning clustering approaches have been put forward to address the HSI clustering task. Most of the existing deep HSI clustering methods can be divided into two stages: high-level feature extraction using deep learning techniques and traditional clustering. In [27], a graph regularized residual subspace clustering network (GR-RSCNet) was presented. Here, the robust nonlinear affinity and deep spectral-spatial representation were learned simultaneously to represent the complex features of HSI within a deep neural network. In [28], Wang et al. devised a scalable graph-based clustering method called SGCNR, which used nonnegative relaxation to represent HSI features. Inspired by the auto-encoder technique in the computer vision domain, some researchers incorporated auto-encoder into the clustering method for spatial-spectral feature learning. For example, Lei et al. [29] designed a spatial-spectral subspace clustering network (DS3C-Net) to extract spatial-spectral features through collaborative constraint and the multi-scale auto-encoder. Hou et al. [30] introduced contrast learning (CC) [31] into HSI feature learning and made use of unlabeled samples to mitigate the problem of insufficient label information. However, the methods aforesaid are not tailored specifically for large-scale HSI clustering, and the clustering performances in complex large-scale HSI dataset clustering need enhancement. Moreover, due to the scarcity of labeled data, extensive spectral variability, and high-dimensionality of HSIs, most of the existing deep clustering methods cannot effectively learn prominent and adaptable high-level features for HSI clustering, leading to low clustering accuracy. Finally, most of the deep clustering methods overlook the layer-wise local features, resulting in poor adaptability to diverse HSI datasets.

To overcome these limitations, we put forward a new self-supervised locality-preserving low-pass graph convolutional embedding approach (L2GCC) for large-scale hyperspectral image clustering. In detail, a spectral-spatial transformation HSI pre-processing mechanism is presented. It aims to learn superpixel-level spectral-spatial features from HSI and cut down the number of graph nodes for the subsequent network processing. Additionally, we create a low-pass graph convolutional embedded autoencoder. This autoencoder learns a hidden representation of the graph by training the inner-product decoder to reconstruct the graph, through which a more smoothed and compact graph representation can be acquired. Moreover, we introduce a layer-wise graph attention module. Its function is to maintain the local features of each layer and enhance the clustering adaptability to various HSI datasets. Finally, we formulate a self-training strategy. In this strategy, a self-training clustering objective utilizes soft labels to monitor the clustering process and get suitable hidden representations for node clustering. In L2GCC, we combine the locality-preserving low-pass graph convolution autoencoder and self-training clustering into a single end-to-end network. By jointly optimizing the loss during network training, they can achieve mutual promotion. In brief, the main contributions of L2GCC are as follows:

- A spectral-spatial transformation HSI pre-processing mechanism is introduced by us. Its purpose is to learn superpixel-level spectral-spatial features from HSI and decrease the quantity of graph nodes for the subsequent network processing.
- We develop a locality-preserving low-pass graph convolutional embedding autoencoder. In this autoencoder, the low-pass graph convolution is crafted to extract smoother features, while the layer-wise graph attention is designed to obtain locality features.
- We put forward a self-training clustering mechanism. This mechanism serves to refine the clustering outcomes and tackle the problem of insufficient labeled samples. Moreover, soft labels derived from graph embedding are proposed to oversee the self-training clustering process.

The locality-preserving low-pass graph convolutional autoencoder and the self-training clustering is jointly incorporated into a single network. They achieve mutual advantage by jointly optimizing the loss. In comparison with the state-of-the-art clustering baselines, the experimental results validate the superiority of our L2GCC.

5.2 Related Work

5.2.1 Notations and Descriptions

In this section, lowercase bold letters are used to represent all vectors, while uppercase letters denote all matrices. We use n, d, and c to stand for the number of nodes, the dimension of HSI (the number of clusters in the node-set $\{x_i\}_{i=1}^{n}$ can be written as

$$\boldsymbol{X} = [x_1, x_2, \ldots, x_n] \in \mathbb{R}^{n \times d} \tag{5.1}$$

Suppose $\mathcal{V}$ represents the set of nodes, $\mathcal{E}$ represents the set of edges among nodes, $\boldsymbol{X} \in \mathbb{R}_{n \times d}$ be the matrix of node features. Then, the graph can be symbolized as $\mathcal{G} = (\mathcal{V}, \mathcal{E})$. Here, the adjacency matrix is indicated by $\boldsymbol{A} \in R_{n \times n}$, and the corresponding degree matrix is shown as $\boldsymbol{D} \in \mathbb{R}_{n \times n}$. Additionally, the operation of concatenation is denoted by $\cdot \| \cdot$. Table 5.1 presents the main notations used in this chapter along with their explanations.

Table 5.1 Main notions and descriptions

Notations	Description
n	Number of nodes contained in the graph
d_i	The dimension of $\boldsymbol{X}$ and the i th latent feature
c	Number of clusters
W	Learnable weight matrix
$\boldsymbol{S}_i$	i th superpixel
$\boldsymbol{X}$	Node feature matrix
$\mathcal{G} = (\mathcal{V}, \mathcal{E})$	Graph $\mathcal{G}$ with edges set $\mathcal{E}$ and nodes set $\mathcal{V}$
$\boldsymbol{A}, \hat{\boldsymbol{A}}_{ij}$	Adjacency matrix of $\mathcal{G}$. The adjacency matrix of a reconstructed graph
$\boldsymbol{D} = \mathrm{diag}(d_1, \ldots, d_n)$	Degree matrix of A
$\boldsymbol{L}, \boldsymbol{L}_{\mathrm{sym}}$	Graph Laplacian Symmetric and normalized Laplacian of $\mathcal{G}$
$\boldsymbol{U}$	Eigenvector matrix of $\boldsymbol{L}_{\mathrm{sym}}$
$\cdot \Vert \cdot$	Concatenation operation
$\boldsymbol{Z}_i$	i th layer encoder output
$\lambda_{\max}, \lambda_i$	Largest eigenvalue, i th eigenvalue
$\mathcal{N}(\cdot)$	Neighborhood of •
$\odot$	Element-wise product
P, Q	The target distribution. The soft labels distribution
η	Learning rate

5.2.2 Convolution on Graph

The graph convolution operation can be interpreted as both spatial operators [32] and spectral operators [33]. In this chapter, we define the convolution operator from the frequency perspective, representing graph signals in the spectral domain. Consider a graph $\mathcal{G} = (\mathcal{V}, \mathcal{E}, \mathbf{A})$, where $\mathcal{V} = \{v_i\}_{i=1,\ldots,n}$ denotes the set of the vertex with n nodes and m channels, $\mathcal{E} = \left\{e_{ij}\right\}_{i,j=1,\ldots,n}$ is the set of edges between nodes (superpixels). The adjacency matrix of the graph is $\boldsymbol{A} \in \mathbb{R}^{n\times n}$, and the weight of the edge between vertex i and vertex j is A_{ij}, in which $A_{ij} = 1, \textit{if} \left\{v_i, v_j\right\} \in \varepsilon$, indicating that there is an edge between node v_i and node v_i; otherwise $A_{ij} = 0$. The node feature matrix is given by $\boldsymbol{X} = \{\boldsymbol{x}_1; \ldots; \boldsymbol{x}_n\}$, where $\boldsymbol{x}_i \in \mathbb{R}^m$ is the feature value associated with node v_i, n represents the number of nodes in the graph, and m is the dimension of i th latent feature. In the graph, we can represent the topological structure of graph $\mathcal{G}$ by constructing an adjacency matrix $\boldsymbol{A}$. The mathematical form of the normalized graph is defined as $\boldsymbol{L} = \boldsymbol{I}_n - \boldsymbol{D}^{-\frac{1}{2}}\boldsymbol{A}\boldsymbol{D}^{-\frac{1}{2}}$, where $\boldsymbol{D}$ is the degree matrix, $\boldsymbol{D}_{ii} = \sum_j \left(\boldsymbol{A}_{i,j}\right)$. $\boldsymbol{L}$ is a real-symmetric positive-semidefinite matrix, and we can factorize $\boldsymbol{L}$ as $\boldsymbol{L} = \boldsymbol{U}\boldsymbol{\Lambda}\boldsymbol{U}^T$, where $\boldsymbol{U} = \left[\boldsymbol{u}_0, \boldsymbol{u}_1, \ldots, \boldsymbol{u}_{n-1}\right] \in \mathbb{R}^{N\times N}$ is the eigenvectors matrix of $\boldsymbol{L}$, that is, $\boldsymbol{U}\boldsymbol{U}^T = \boldsymbol{E}$ with $\boldsymbol{E}$ being the identity matrix, and $\boldsymbol{\Lambda}$ is the diagonal matrix of eigenvalues with $\boldsymbol{\Lambda}_{ii} = \boldsymbol{\lambda}_i$, $\boldsymbol{\lambda}_i$ denotes the eigenvalue. Given a graph signal

$X \in \mathbb{R}^N$ (graph node feature vector), the Fourier transform of X is expressed as $\mathcal{F}(X) = U^T X$, and the inverse graph Fourier transform is $\mathcal{F}^{-1}(\hat{X}) = U\hat{X}$, where $\hat{X}$ is the result of the Fourier transform. The graph Fourier transform projects the graph feature vector into an orthogonal space whose basis is composed of the eigenvectors of the normalized graph Laplace operator. The elements in $\hat{X}$ are the coordinates of X projected into the orthogonal space, and X can be written as $X = \sum_i \hat{x}_i u_i$. The graph convolution of X with a graph filter g can be expressed as

$$\begin{aligned} g * X &= \mathcal{F}^{-1}(F(x) \odot F(g)) \\ &= U\left(U^T X \odot U^T g\right) \end{aligned} \tag{5.2}$$

If the graph filter is expressed as $g_\theta = \mathrm{diag}(U^T g)$, then the Eq. (5.2) can be simplified as

$$g_\theta * X = U g_\theta(\Lambda) U^{\mathrm{T}} X \tag{5.3}$$

All spectral-based graph convolution algorithms adhere to the definition given in Eq. (5.3). In spectral-based graph convolution algorithms, the graph filter holds great significance. The design of the graph filter has the ability to decide the performances of these algorithms. The aggregation operation within GCN is presented as follows:

$$X_{i+1} = \sigma\left(D^{-\frac{1}{2}} \hat{A} D^{-\frac{1}{2}} X_i W_i\right) \tag{5.4}$$

5.2.3 *Attention Convolution on Graph*

For a given graph $\mathcal{G}$, the feature eigenvector of every node is $x_i \in \mathbb{R}^m$. By applying a linear transformation to x_i, a new eigenvector $x_i' \in \mathbb{R}^{m'}$ can be derived. The operation procedure can be written as

$$x_i' = W x_i,\ W \in \mathbb{R}^{m \times m'} \tag{5.5}$$

When node j is a neighbor of node i, the attention mechanism can be utilized to compute the significance of node j with respect to node i. The attention score e_{ij} is calculated in the following way

$$e_{ij} = \left(\sigma\left(a^T\left[W x_i || W x_j\right]\right)\right) \tag{5.6}$$

where $||$ represents the concatenation operation. The parameter vector $a^T \in \mathbb{R}^{2m'}$, and σ stands for a nonlinear layer, specifically, *LeakyReLU*.

The value of e_{ij} can be transformed into the subsequent form by means of a softmax function

$$\alpha_{ij} = \text{softmax}(e_{ij}) = \frac{\exp\left(\sigma\left(\boldsymbol{a}^T\left[\mathbf{W}\boldsymbol{x}_i||\mathbf{W}\boldsymbol{x}_j\right]\right)\right)}{\sum_{k\in N_i}\exp\left(\sigma\left(\boldsymbol{a}^T\left[\mathbf{W}\boldsymbol{x}_i||\mathbf{W}\boldsymbol{x}_j\right]\right)\right)} \tag{5.7}$$

The mathematical expression of graph convolution output of GAT is

$$\boldsymbol{x}_i' = \sigma\left(\sum_{j\in n_i}\alpha_{ij}\cdot\mathbf{W}^T\boldsymbol{x}_j\right) \tag{5.8}$$

where σ serves as the activation function. a_{ij} represents the learned attention weight, and n_i indicates the quantity of neighbor nodes of node i.

5.2.4 Graph Auto-encoder

The graph autoencoder (GAE) [34] makes use of multi-layer GCN to acquire the hidden representation of graph node embeddings. It computes the inner-products between pairs of nodes, maps them into a probability space using a sigmoid function to calculate similarities, and then reconstructs the graph by calculating the graph reconstruction loss. The network architectures of GAEs in [34–37] usually exhibit asymmetry. However, we can use graph sharpening to design a symmetric architecture. For example, in the Adversarial Regularized Graph Auto-Encoder [37], adversarial learning is integrated into GAE to boost its robustness. In the GAE with Adaptive Graph Convolution [36], a high-order convolution operator is introduced to GAE to enhance its representation ability.

5.3 Proposed Method

5.3.1 Problem Definition and Overall Framework

Given an undirected graph $\mathcal{G}$, the objective is to categorize the nodes into c clusters, namely $\{C_1, C_2, \ldots, C_c\}$, by leveraging a self-supervised locality-preserving low-pass graph convolutional embedding auto-encoder to learn the latent representation $\boldsymbol{Z}$. As a result, nodes within a single cluster possess similar spectral feature values and spatial structures.

Based on the flow-diagram of L2GCC in Fig. 5.1, our method can be divided into three segments: pixel-to-region transformation, locality-preserving low-pass graph convolutional embedding encoder, and graph convolution embedding decoder.

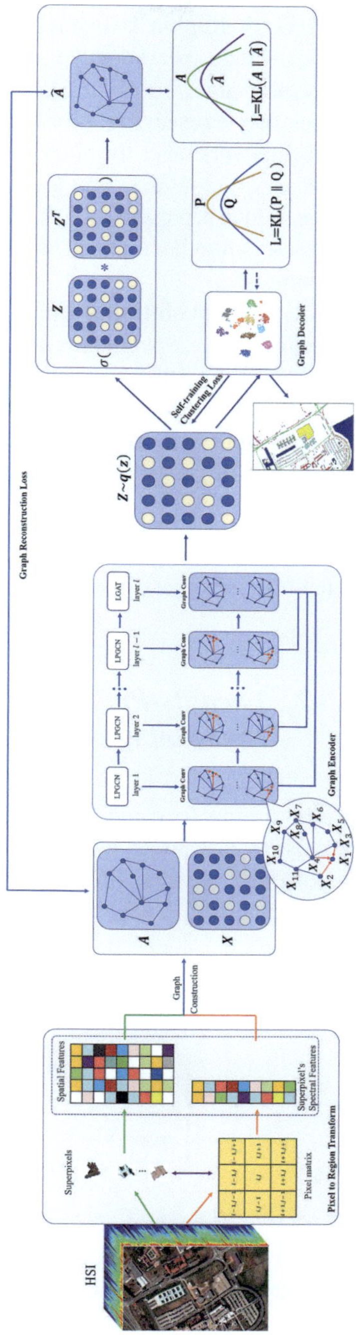

Fig. 5.1 We depicts the flow-diagram of the proposed hyperspectral image clustering network featuring self-supervised locality-preserving low-pass graph convolutional embedding (L2GCC). At first, the HSI is converted into graph nodes via the pixel-to-region transformation module. After that, the adjacency matrix $\boldsymbol{A}$ is computed and the graph is built. Next, a locality-preserving low-pass graph convolutional embedding autoencoder is used to learn the hidden representation $\boldsymbol{Z}$. In this autoencoder, the low-pass GCN is designed to extract smoother features, and the layer-wise GAT is for extracting locality features. Eventually, self-training clustering is carried out, and the weights are updated by jointly optimizing the loss during network training

- **Pixel-To-Region Transformation**: The HSI is divided into local superpixels, and the average spectral value of the pixels within each superpixel is regarded as the feature value.
- **Locality-Preserving Low-Pass Graph Convolutional Embedding Encoder**: The network takes the node feature and the graph structure as inputs. The locality-preserving low-pass graph convolutional embedding autoencoder is used to learn the hidden representation $\boldsymbol{Z}$. In this autoencoder, the low-pass GCN is intended to extract smoother features, while the layer-wise GAT is designed to extract locality features.
- **Graph Convolutional Embedding Decoder**: The proposed approach includes two decoders. Specifically, the graph is reconstructed by minimizing the KL divergence between the distribution of the adjacency matrix $\boldsymbol{A}$ and that of the adjacency matrix $\hat{\boldsymbol{A}}$ of the reconstructed graph. Moreover, self-training clustering can be carried out by minimizing the KL divergence between the target distribution $\boldsymbol{P}$ and the distribution $\boldsymbol{Q}$ of the soft labels.

The HSI preprocessing, graph convolutional embedding autoencoder, and node clustering are integrated into a unified network, where each component provides benefits to the others. Thus, the proposed network is an end-to-end training network.

5.3.2 Locality-Preserving Low-Pass Graph Convolutional Embedding Encoder

When aiming to categorize graph nodes into various clusters, the fundamental premise is that nodes within the same cluster ought to be highly related. In other words, they possess similar spatial-spectral characteristics. As a result, the latent representation $\boldsymbol{Z}$ is expected to be smooth across the graph manifold.

Assumption 1 In an ideal scenario, the intra-cluster distance is minimized while the inter-cluster distance is maximized, that is

$$\begin{cases} \min \sum_{i=1}^{m} \sum_{j=1}^{m} d(i,j) = \min \sum_{i=1}^{m} \sum_{j=1}^{m} f(\boldsymbol{x}_i) - f(\boldsymbol{x}_j)_2^2 \\ \max \sum_{\alpha=1}^{c} \sum_{\beta=1}^{c} d(\alpha,\beta) = \max \sum_{\alpha=1}^{c} \sum_{\beta=1}^{c} y(\boldsymbol{c}_\alpha) - y(\boldsymbol{c}_\beta)_2^2 \end{cases} \tag{5.9}$$

where $\boldsymbol{x}_i$ represents the node feature corresponding to node i. The mapping $f(\cdot)$ is designed to extract the optimal spatial-spectral representation of the node. m denotes the quantity of nodes within a cluster. The function $y(\cdot)$ is used to compute the central feature of the cluster, and c is the number of clusters (classes).

1. *Low-pass Graph Convolutional Filter:* A graph signal (node feature) can be considered smooth when the representations of neighboring nodes on the graph have similar features. For a given graph signal $\boldsymbol{X}$, we are able to assess the

smoothness of the graph signal $\boldsymbol{X}$ by calculating the Rayleigh quotient [38], which is

$$R(\boldsymbol{L}, \boldsymbol{X}) = \frac{\boldsymbol{X}^\top \boldsymbol{L} \boldsymbol{X}}{\boldsymbol{X}^\top \boldsymbol{X}} = \frac{\sum_{(x_i, x_j) \in \mathcal{E}} (x_i - x_j)^2}{\sum_{i \in v} x_i^2} \tag{5.10}$$

where $\boldsymbol{L}$ stands for the graph Laplacian, and x_i is the feature of the i-th node. As shown in Eq. (5.10), smooth signals are expected to have comparable values on adjacent nodes, and signals with greater smoothness have a lower Rayleigh quotient.

Theorem 1 *Smoother signals can be achieved by filtering out high-frequency basis signals and retaining low-frequency basis signals.*

Based on the principle of Theorem 1, we can devise a low-pass graph filter to handle the graph signals for node clustering. There are multiple ways to represent a low-pass graph filter. In this chapter, the frequency response function of the low-pass graph filter is

$$p(\lambda_i) = 1 - k\lambda_i \tag{5.11}$$

where k represents a real numerical value, and λ_i signifies the ith eigenvalue. By referring to the frequency response function $p(\cdot)$ in Eq. (5.11), the mathematical representation of the graph filter $\boldsymbol{G}$ is given as

$$\boldsymbol{G} = \boldsymbol{U} p(\boldsymbol{\Lambda}) \boldsymbol{U}^{-1} = \boldsymbol{U}(\boldsymbol{I} - k\boldsymbol{\Lambda})\boldsymbol{U}^{-1} = \boldsymbol{I} - k\boldsymbol{L} \tag{5.12}$$

Theorem 2 *Provided a graph filter* $\mathbf{G}$, *when its frequency–response function* $p(\lambda)$ *is non-negative and non-increasing for every* λ_i, *then for any given signal* $\boldsymbol{X}$ *and the filtered version* $\tilde{\boldsymbol{X}} = \boldsymbol{G}\boldsymbol{X}$, *we will always get.*

$$R(\tilde{\boldsymbol{X}}, \boldsymbol{X}) \leq R(\boldsymbol{L}, \boldsymbol{X}) \tag{5.13}$$

Based on Theorem 2, when such a low-pass graph filter is used on a graph signal, the filtered node features have similar feature values in each dimension. This makes subsequent network clustering easier. By conducting graph convolution on the node feature matrix $\boldsymbol{X}$**,** the filtered feature $\tilde{\boldsymbol{X}}$ can be derived as

$$\tilde{\boldsymbol{X}} = \boldsymbol{G}\boldsymbol{X} = \boldsymbol{U} p(\boldsymbol{\Lambda}) \boldsymbol{U}^{-1} \cdot \boldsymbol{U} \boldsymbol{p} = \sum_{i=1}^{n} (1 - k\lambda_i) c_i \boldsymbol{u}_i = \sum_{i=1}^{n} c_i^{'} \boldsymbol{u}_i \tag{5.14}$$

where $\tilde{\boldsymbol{X}} = [\tilde{\boldsymbol{x}}_1, \tilde{\boldsymbol{x}}_2, \ldots, \tilde{\boldsymbol{x}}_n]^T$, c_i is the coefficient of i-th eigenvector $\boldsymbol{u}_i$.

Moreover, the l-order graph convolution is formulated as

$$\tilde{\boldsymbol{X}} = (\boldsymbol{I} - k\boldsymbol{L})^l \boldsymbol{X} = \tilde{\boldsymbol{G}} \boldsymbol{X} \tag{5.15}$$

In Eq. (5.15), the filter of the l-order graph convolution is $\tilde{\boldsymbol{G}} = (I - k\boldsymbol{L})^l$, and its frequency-response function is

$$p(\lambda_q) = (1 - k\lambda_q)^l \tag{5.16}$$

In actual use, the graph Laplacian $\boldsymbol{L}$ is frequently normalized to be as follows

$$\tilde{\boldsymbol{L}}_{\text{sym}} = \tilde{\boldsymbol{D}}^{-\frac{1}{2}}\tilde{\boldsymbol{L}}\tilde{\boldsymbol{D}}^{-\frac{1}{2}} = \tilde{\boldsymbol{U}}\tilde{\boldsymbol{\Lambda}}\tilde{\boldsymbol{U}}^{-1} \tag{5.17}$$

Here, the Laplacian matrix and degree matrix corresponding to $\tilde{\boldsymbol{A}} = \boldsymbol{I} + \boldsymbol{A}$ are denoted as $\tilde{\boldsymbol{L}}$ and $\tilde{\boldsymbol{D}}$ respectively. After that, $\tilde{\boldsymbol{\Lambda}}$ represents the decomposition of $\tilde{\boldsymbol{L}}_{\text{sym}}$. Then the filter can be expressed as

$$\boldsymbol{G} = I - k\tilde{\boldsymbol{L}}_{\text{sym}} \tag{5.18}$$

It's important to note that when k is set at 1, the graph filter becomes the traditional GCN filter. Equation (5.18) presents the concept of devising a low-pass convolution kernel. Nevertheless, varying k values will result in distinct performances of the low-pass filter. With reference to the proof of Theorem 1 and Eq. (5.17), the smoothness of the filtered graph signal $\tilde{\boldsymbol{X}}$ can be gauged by

$$R(\boldsymbol{L}, \tilde{\boldsymbol{X}}) = \frac{\tilde{\boldsymbol{X}}^\top \boldsymbol{L}\tilde{\boldsymbol{X}}}{\tilde{\boldsymbol{X}}^\top \tilde{\boldsymbol{X}}} = \frac{\sum_{i=1}^n g_i \lambda_i}{\sum_{i=1}^n g_i} \tag{5.19}$$

where $g_i > 0$ serves as a coefficient. For getting a smoother filter, g_i ought to decline as λ_i grows. The maximum eigenvalue is symbolized as $\lambda_{\max}$. In theory, if $k > 1/\lambda_{\max}$, the graph filter is not low-pass since g_i rises in the interval $(1/k, \lambda_{\max})$. Yet, when $k < 1/\lambda_{\max}$, not all high-frequency basis signals can be filtered. Thus, the optimal value for k is $1/\lambda_{\max}$.

Based on the propagation rules of GCN, the propagation function of a low-pass graph convolutional network is constructed as

$$\boldsymbol{Z}_{l+1} = \phi\left(\tilde{\boldsymbol{D}}^{\frac{1}{2}}\tilde{\boldsymbol{A}}\tilde{\boldsymbol{D}}^{-\frac{1}{2}}\boldsymbol{Z}_l\boldsymbol{W}^{(l)}\right) \tag{5.20}$$

where the learned representation of the l-th layer is denoted as $\boldsymbol{Z}_l$, and $\boldsymbol{Z}_0 = \boldsymbol{X}$. Meanwhile, $\boldsymbol{W}^{(l)}$ is the coefficient matrix learned in the process of network training.

2. *Layer-wise Graph Attention Module (LGAT):* As mentioned earlier, one can design a low-pass graph convolutional filter by filtering out high-frequency basis signals while retaining low-frequency basis signals. Nevertheless, the low-pass GCN is unable to learn layer-specific intermediate information for node clustering. Moreover, existing deep clustering methods typically focus only on global refinement and overlook the multi-scale spatial-spectral features hidden

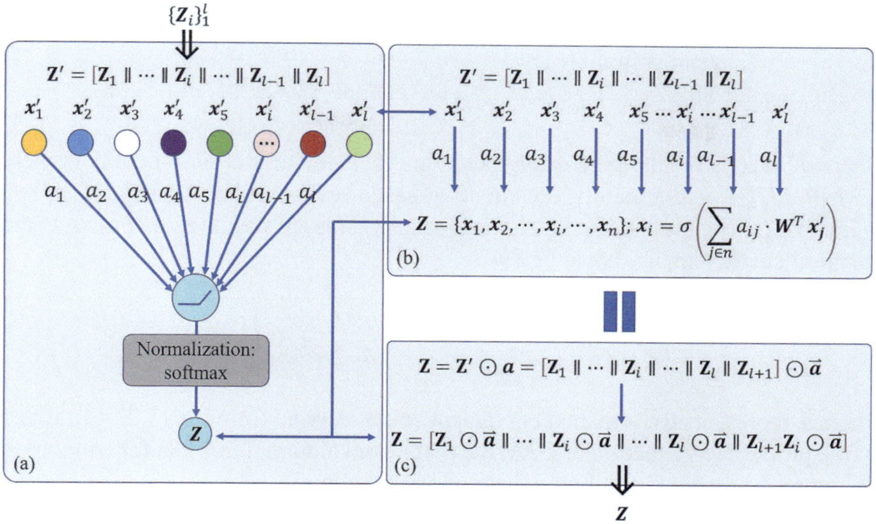

Fig. 5.2 Conceptual depictions of the suggested layer-by-layer graph attention (LGAT) module are as follows. In **a**, it shows the visual chart of LGAT. For **b**, the multi-scale layer-wise local information is retained through a concatenation approach, and then LGAT is demonstrated from a node-by-node viewpoint. In **c**, we explain the mechanism of LGAT from a layer-by-layer aspect. Here, the 'softmax' represents the softmax function for normalization. We use "⇓" to indicate the input and output of LGAT

in different layers [39]. To solve these problems and make use of the multi-scale layer-wise local information, we develop the LGAT module.

Features at various layers offer different degrees of semantic descriptions to represent the input data, and the final clustering task might demand different layer-wise local information. A conceptual visual explanation is presented in Fig. 5.2.

Since distinct layers possess diverse spectral dimensions, initially, we maintain the multi-scale layer-wise local information in a concatenation style, that is

$$\boldsymbol{Z}' = \left[\mathbf{Z}_1 \| \ldots \|\mathbf{Z}_i\| \ldots \|\mathbf{Z}_l\|\mathbf{Z}_{l+1}\right] \tag{5.21}$$

where l denotes the graph convolutional layer. $\mathbf{Z}_i \in \mathbb{R}^{n\times d_i}$ represents the graph feature representations of the i th layer, having a dimension of d_i. Specifically, $\boldsymbol{Z}' = \left\{\boldsymbol{x}'_1, \boldsymbol{x}'_2, \ldots, \boldsymbol{x}'_n\right\} \in \mathbb{R}^{n\times d_z}$, where $z = \sum_{i=1}^{l} d_i$, $\boldsymbol{x}'_2$ is the node feature vector following the concatenation operation.

Afterward, we utilize the graph attention mechanism to extract the concatenated features $\boldsymbol{Z}'$. The attention coefficient a_{ij} between node i and node j can be expressed as

$$\alpha_{ij} = \text{softmax}\left(e_{ij}\right) = \frac{\exp\left(\sigma\left(\boldsymbol{a}^T\left[\boldsymbol{W}\boldsymbol{x}_i'||\boldsymbol{W}\boldsymbol{x}_j'\right]\right)\right)}{\sum_{j\in n}\exp\left(\sigma\left(\boldsymbol{a}^T\left[\boldsymbol{W}\boldsymbol{x}_i'||\boldsymbol{W}\boldsymbol{x}_j'\right]\right)\right)} \tag{5.22}$$

where $\boldsymbol{a}^T$ stands for the parameter vector, and σ is the activation function, namely $LeakyReLU(\cdot)$. Subsequently, the attention-based scale-by-scale strategy is applied to Eq. (5.21). The multi-scale layer-wise local features are weighted according to the attention coefficient, as shown below.

$$\begin{aligned} Z = \boldsymbol{Z}' \odot a &= \left[\boldsymbol{Z}_1\| \ldots \|\boldsymbol{Z}_i\| \ldots \|\boldsymbol{Z}_l\|\boldsymbol{Z}_{l+1}\right] \odot \vec{\boldsymbol{\alpha}} \\ &= \left[\boldsymbol{Z}_1 \odot \vec{\boldsymbol{\alpha}}\| \ldots \|\boldsymbol{Z}_i \odot \vec{\boldsymbol{\alpha}}\| \ldots \|\boldsymbol{Z}_l \odot \vec{\boldsymbol{\alpha}}\|\boldsymbol{Z}_{l+1} \odot \vec{\boldsymbol{\alpha}}\right] \end{aligned} \tag{5.23}$$

where $\vec{\boldsymbol{\alpha}}$ represents the attention coefficient vector derived from Eq. (5.22). Drawing on the propagation function of GAT, the graph convolutional formula for computing the output features of each individual node is as follows

$$\boldsymbol{x}_i = \sigma\left(\sum_{j\in n}\alpha_{ij}\cdot\boldsymbol{W}^T\boldsymbol{x}_j'\right) \tag{5.24}$$

Based on Eq. (5.23), we observe that $\boldsymbol{x}_i$ encompasses abundant layer-by-layer information for various clustering tasks.

5.3.3 Graph Convolutional Embedding Decoder

In the method we put forward, we create decoders, specifically the graph reconstruction decoder and the graph convolutional embedding clustering decoder, to decipher the hidden representation $\boldsymbol{Z}$ learned by the locality-preserving low-pass graph convolutional embedding encoder and to modify the trainable weight of L2GCC.

1. *Graph Reconstruction Decoder:* In our proposed approach, in order to reconstruct both the node features and the graph structure, a straightforward inner-product decoder is utilized to represent the reconstructed adjacency matrix, that is

$$\hat{\boldsymbol{A}}_{ij} = \text{sigmoid}\left(\boldsymbol{Z}^\top\boldsymbol{Z}\right) \tag{5.25}$$

where $\hat{\boldsymbol{A}}_{ij}$ represents the adjacency matrix of the reconstructed graph. This matrix is both flexible and efficient in portraying the structure of the reconstructed graph. By using this method, we are able to decode the content and structure of the initial graph. To gauge the disparity between the reconstructed graph adjacency matrix $\hat{\boldsymbol{A}}$ and the original graph adjacency matrix $\boldsymbol{A}$, we make use of Kullback–Leibler (KL) Divergence to measure the difference between the two distributions. The graph reconstruction loss is expressed as

$$L_r = \mathrm{KL}\big(\boldsymbol{A} \| \hat{\boldsymbol{A}}\big) \tag{5.26}$$

2. *Graph Convolutional Embedding Self-Training Clustering Decoder:* As previously stated, a locality-preserving low-pass graph convolutional embedding autoencoder can be used to learn a graph hidden representation $\mathbf{Z}$. Nevertheless, clustering is not involved in the autoencoder procedure, and it is simplistic to dissociate clustering from embedding learning since the learned $\mathbf{Z}$ might not be suitable for clustering. Additionally, a major obstacle in unsupervised graph clustering is the lack of labels for training the network. To address these issues, taking inspiration from DEC [42], we devise a self-training strategy. In this strategy, the self-training clustering objective utilizes soft labels to oversee the clustering process and acquire suitable hidden representations for node clustering. The self-training clustering loss is expressed as

$$L_c = \mathrm{KL}(P \| Q) = \sum_i \sum_j p_{ij} \log \frac{p_{ij}}{q_{ij}} \tag{5.27}$$

where $\mathrm{KL}(\cdot \| \cdot)$ denotes the Kullback–Leibler divergence. p_{ij} represents the target distribution, and Q is the soft labels distribution. We are able to use q_{ij} to gauge the similarity between the cluster center μ_j and the node embedding z_i of node i. This similarity is measured by a Student's t-distribution, that is

$$q_{ij} = \frac{\left(1 + z_i - \mu_j^2\right)^{-1}}{\sum_{j'} \left(1 + z_i - \mu_{j'}^2\right)^{-1}} \tag{5.28}$$

We can regard each node as a soft clustering assignment distribution. Moreover, we define the target distribution p_{ij} as follows

$$p_{ij} = \frac{q_{ij}^2 / \sum_i q_{ij}}{\sum_k \left(q_{ik}^2 / \sum_i q_{ik}\right)} \tag{5.29}$$

where $\sum_i q_{ij}$ is a normalization factor used to standardize the loss contribution of each centroid and avoid the distortion of the hidden feature space caused by large clusters.

As mentioned earlier, a more concentrated Q distribution can be achieved by minimizing L_c. That is to say, it makes the nodes within the same class more alike in distribution and increases the distance between nodes from different classes. In this manner, we can convert unsupervised clustering into "semi-supervised" clustering.

5.3.4 Joint Embedding and Optimization

In the methodology we've developed, L2GCC is optimized through the combination of the graph-embedded autoencoder and self-training clustering. Subsequently, the overall objective function can be defined as

$$L = L_r + \gamma L_c \tag{5.30}$$

where L_r represents the reconstruction loss of the graph autoencoder as presented in Eq. (5.26). L_c is the self-training clustering loss defined in Eq. (5.27). The coefficient weight $\gamma \geq 0$ is utilized to regulate the degree of distortion in the embedded space. In our approach, γ is set to 0.1.

In the L2GCC, we need to update three parameters using Gradient Descent. These parameters are the coefficient weight $W^{(l)}$, the cluster center μ_j, and the target distribution p_{ij}.

- **Updating the weights and cluster centers.** When p_{ij} is fixed, the gradient of L_c with respect to μ_j can be written as

$$\frac{\partial L_c}{\partial \mu_j} = 2\sum_{i=1}^{N}\left(1 + z_i - \mu_j^2\right)^{-1}(q_{ij} - p_{ij})(z_i - \mu_j) \tag{5.31}$$

  Given a learning rate η, we can update the μ_j by

$$\mu_j = \mu_j - \eta\frac{\partial L_c}{\partial \mu_j} \tag{5.32}$$

  Then the coefficient weight $W^{(l)}$ is updated by

$$W^{(l)} = W^{(l)} - \eta\left(\frac{\partial L_r}{\partial W^{(l)}} + \gamma\frac{\partial L_c}{\partial W^{(l)}}\right) \tag{5.33}$$

- **Updating the target distribution.** During the training phase, the target distribution p_{ij} can be regarded as "ground-truth labels". It needs to be updated every T iterations using all the embedded nodes. The m initial centroids $\{\mu_j\}_{j=1}^{m}$ are derived by performing k-means clustering on the embedded nodes $\mathbf{Z}$. Subsequently, p_{ij} is updated according to Eqs. (5.28) and (5.29), and the label of n_i can be estimated with

$$n_i = arg\, \underset{j}{max}\, q_{ij} \tag{5.34}$$

For this purpose, initially, the L2GCC autoencoder is trained without self-training clustering. As detailed in Sect. 3.2, this is done to learn a good representation $\mathbf{Z}$.

Subsequently, self-training clustering is carried out to enhance the embedding. The training process will be halted when the change in the target distribution p_{ij} between two successive updates is smaller than a fixed δ or when the number of training epochs T reaches the pre-set upper limit. The clustering outcome is given by the last optimized soft labels distribution Q. The training procedure of the proposed L2GCC is depicted in Algorithm 1.

Algorithm 1: L2GCC training process

Input: Graph $\mathcal{G}$; Number of initial centroids m; Number of iterations T; Coefficient weight γ; Distribution threshold δ.
Output: Clustering results Q.
Initialization: $t = 1$; $\boldsymbol{Z}^{(0)} = \boldsymbol{X}$; Initialize the parameters of graph autoencoder;
Calculate graph Laplacian $\tilde{\boldsymbol{L}}_{\text{sym}}$ by Eq. (5.17);
$k \leftarrow 1/\lambda_{\max}$;
Get the graph hidden presentation $\boldsymbol{Z}$ by performing graph autoencoder according to minimizing Eq. (5.26);
Get m initial clusters centroid μ_j by k-means clustering based on $\boldsymbol{Z}$
for $t = 1$ to $T - 1$ do
    The soft labels distribution Q is calculated based on μ and $\boldsymbol{Z}$ by Eq. (5.28);
    The target distribution P is calculated based on Q by Eq. (5.29);
    The self-training clustering loss L_c is calculated by Eq. (5.27);
    if $L_c \leq \delta$ **break**;
    Calculate joint embedding loss L by Eq. (5.30) and update the weight matrices adopting Adam gradient descent;
end
Obtain the final clustering results Q according to Eq. (5.34)

5.3.5 *HSI Pre-processing and Graph Construction*

HSI encompasses abundant spectral details and a vast number of pixels. This not only offers ample features for target classification but also results in a substantial computational load. In practical scenarios, the computational complexity of a graph convolutional neural network (GNN) escalates exponentially as the number of nodes grows. Calculating each pixel as a graph node is infeasible. Put differently, the key issue in HSI pre-processing is how to decrease the number of nodes while maintaining the hyperspectral spectral-spatial traits. To build a graph that can be clustered by the subsequent network, we present an HSI pre-processing approach. This approach consists of two components: a spatial transformer and a spectral transformer.

- **Spatial transformer:** Suppose we have an HSI cube $I_B = \{x_1, x_2, \ldots, x_m\}$ with $m = \mathcal{W} \times \mathcal{H}$ pixels and $\mathcal{B}$ spectral bands, where w, $\mathcal{H}$ stand for the width and height respectively. First, we use unsupervised PCA [40] to lower the dimensionality of the HSI. We keep the first principal component to create a reduced image $I_b = \{x_1^r, x_2^r, \ldots, x_m^r\}$. After that, we apply the SLIC [41] to group the pixels into superpixels. The mathematical expression of a local superpixel can be defined as

$$HSI = \bigcup_{i=1}^{K} \mathcal{S}_i, \mathcal{S}_i \cap \mathcal{S}_j = \emptyset, i \neq j; i, j = 1, 2, \ldots, K \tag{5.35}$$

where $\mathcal{S}_i = \{p_{i,1}, \ldots, p_{i,n_i}\}$ represents a superpixel that consists of n_i connected pixels, and K is the overall quantity of superpixels.

- **Spectral transformer:** As indicated previously, the spatial transformer enables us to divide the HSI into superpixels. Nevertheless, the dimensionality reduction process causes the loss of the HSI's spectral information. In other words, the superpixel fails to comprehensively extract the spectral features of the HSI. To address this issue, we directly extract the spectral value of each pixel from the original HSI. Subsequently, we calculate the average spectral value of the pixels within a superpixel, which serves as the superpixel's spectral feature. The spectral feature vector of the pixel at the spatial location $p_0 = (x, y)$ can be written as

$$\boldsymbol{x}(\boldsymbol{p}_0) = (X_1(\boldsymbol{p}_0), X_2(\boldsymbol{p}_0), \ldots, X_{\mathcal{B}}(\boldsymbol{p}_0)) \tag{5.36}$$

where $X_i(\boldsymbol{p}_0)$ represents the spectral value of the pixel in the i th channel at the spatial location $\boldsymbol{p}_0$.

Subsequently, the mathematical formula for the HSI feature $\boldsymbol{X}$ is

$$X = [\boldsymbol{X}_1, \boldsymbol{X}_2, \ldots \boldsymbol{X}_S]^T = \left[\frac{1}{\tau_1}\sum_{k=1}^{N_1} \boldsymbol{x}\frac{1}{k}, \frac{1}{\tau_2}\sum_{k=1}^{N_2} \boldsymbol{x}\frac{2}{k}, \ldots, \frac{1}{\tau_k}\sum_{k=1}^{N_1} \boldsymbol{x}\frac{S}{k}\right]^T \tag{5.37}$$

where $\boldsymbol{X}_i$ is the feature vector of the ith superpixel, and τ_i indicates the number of pixels within the superpixel. $\boldsymbol{x}_k^i$ is the spectral feature vector of the pixel, as presented in Eq. (5.36).

- **Graph construction:** In our proposed approach, we utilize superpixels as the nodes of the graph. The adjacency matrix $\boldsymbol{A}$, which determines the connections between vertices, is commonly calculated via a radial basis function (RBF).

$$\boldsymbol{A}_{ij} = \begin{cases} e^{-\rho \boldsymbol{X}_i - \boldsymbol{X}_j^2}, & \text{if } \boldsymbol{X}_i \in \mathcal{N}_t(\boldsymbol{X}_j) \text{ or } \boldsymbol{X}_j \in \mathcal{N}_t(\boldsymbol{X}_i) \\ 0, & \text{otherwise} \end{cases} \tag{5.38}$$

where $\rho = 0.2$ is an empirical set to control the RBF's width, $\boldsymbol{X}_i$ denote nodes features of nodes i, $\mathcal{N}_t(\boldsymbol{X}_i)$ is the t-hop neighbors of $\boldsymbol{X}_i$.

5.3.6 Computational Complexity

Let n denote the quantity of graph nodes, d the spectral dimension of the input nodes, d_i the spectral dimension of nodes in the ith layer, $|\mathcal{E}|$ the number of non-zero entries in the adjacency matrix A, c be the number of clusters, l be the number of graphs embedded auto-encoder layers. The computational complexity of low-pass GCN convolution is estimated as $O\left[(n+|\mathcal{E}|)\left(dd_1+\sum_{i=2}^{l-1} d_i d_{i-1}\right)\right]$. For layer-wise GAT, the computational complexity is $O\left[|\mathcal{E}|\left(\sum_{i=1}^{l-1} d_i\right)d_l\right]$. The computational complexity of graph auto-encoder is $O\left[(n+|\mathcal{E}|)\left(dd_1+\sum_{i=2}^{l-1} d_i d_{i-1}\right)+|\mathcal{E}|\left(\sum_{i=1}^{l-1} d_i\right)d_l\right]$. For Eq. (5.29), the computational complexity is $O\left[(nc+n\log n)+\left(n^2+n\log n\right)\right]$. Therefore, the computational complexity of performing clustering on the graph in each iteration is $O\left[(n+|\mathcal{E}|)\left(dd_1+\sum_{i=2}^{l-1} d_i d_{i-1}\right)+|\mathcal{E}|\left(\sum_{i=1}^{l-1} d_i\right)d_l + (nc+n\ \log\ n)+\left(n^2+n\ \log\ n\right)\right]$. If our model iterates T times, we express the overall computational complexity of LGCC is $O\left[\left[(n+|\mathrm{E}|)\left(dd_1+\sum_{i=2}^{l-1} d_i d_{i-1}\right)+|\mathrm{E}|\left(\sum_{i=1}^{l-1} d_i\right) d_l+(nc+n\ \log\ n)+\left(n^2+n\ \log\ n\right)\right]T\right]$ From the formula for computational complexity, we can significantly decrease the computational complexity by reducing the number of nodes. This validates the effectiveness of the HSI pre-processing.

5.4 Proof

Theorem 1 *Smoother signals can be acquired by keeping low-frequency basis signals and filtering high-frequency ones.*

Proof When we have a graph signal (node features) $\boldsymbol{X}$, by considering $\boldsymbol{L}=\boldsymbol{U}\boldsymbol{\Lambda}\boldsymbol{U}^{-1}$ and referring to Eq. (5.10), we can describe the smoothness of the eigenvector $\boldsymbol{u}_{\mathrm{q}}$ smoothness as

$$R(\boldsymbol{L},\boldsymbol{u}_q)=\frac{\boldsymbol{u}_q^{\top}\boldsymbol{L}\boldsymbol{u}_q}{\boldsymbol{u}_q^{\top}\boldsymbol{u}_q}=\lambda_q \tag{5.39}$$

where $\boldsymbol{u}_q(i)$ is the $\boldsymbol{u}_q$'s i-th element. Equation (5.39) indicates that eigenvectors with better smoothness possess smaller eigenvalues. Subsequently, we can break down $\boldsymbol{X}$ into a linear combination, that is

$$\boldsymbol{X}=\boldsymbol{U}\boldsymbol{c}=\sum_{q=1}^{n} c_q\boldsymbol{u}_q \tag{5.40}$$

where c_q represents the coefficient of the q-th eigenvector $\boldsymbol{u}_q$. Therefore, the smoothness of $\boldsymbol{X}$ can be computed according to Eqs. (5.10), (5.39), and (5.40)

$$R(\boldsymbol{L}, \boldsymbol{X}) = \frac{\boldsymbol{X}^\top \boldsymbol{L}\boldsymbol{X}}{\boldsymbol{X}^\top \boldsymbol{X}} = \frac{\sum_{c=1}^{n} c_q^2 \lambda_c}{\sum_{c=1}^{n} c_q^2} \tag{5.41}$$

Therefore, the Theorem 1 is proved.

Theorem 2 *Provided with a graph filter* $\mathbf{G}$, *in the case where its frequency response function* $p(\lambda)$ *is non-negative and non-increasing for every* λ_i, *then for any given signal* $\boldsymbol{X}$ *and the filtered* $\tilde{\boldsymbol{X}} = \boldsymbol{G}\boldsymbol{X}$, *it is always true that*

$$R\big(\tilde{\boldsymbol{X}}, \boldsymbol{X}\big) \leq R(\boldsymbol{L}, \boldsymbol{X}) \tag{5.42}$$

Namely

$$\frac{\sum_{i=1}^{n} b_i \lambda_i}{\sum_{i=1}^{n} b_i} \leq \frac{\sum_{i=1}^{n} c_i \lambda_i}{\sum_{i=1}^{n} c_i} \tag{5.43}$$

Proof We adopt induction to prove the Theorem 2, namely.

$$R_b^i = \frac{\sum_{i=1}^{n} b_i \lambda_i}{\sum_{i=1}^{n} b_i} \tag{5.44}$$

$$R_c^i = \frac{\sum_{i=1}^{n} c_i \lambda_i}{\sum_{i=1}^{n} c_i}$$

If, $\lambda_1 \leq \dots \lambda_n$, and $\frac{c_1}{b_1} \leq \dots \leq \frac{c_n}{b_n}$, we can easily prove that $R_b^2 \leq R_c^2$. Now, suppose that $n = l - 1$, and $R_b^{l-1} \leq R_c^{l-1}$, then we have R_b^l

$$\begin{aligned} \frac{\sum_{i=1}^{l} b_i \lambda_i}{\sum_{i=1}^{l} b_i} &= \frac{\sum_{i=1}^{l-1} b_i \lambda_i + b_l \lambda_l}{\sum_{i=1}^{l-1} b_i + b_l} \\ &= \frac{\left(\sum_{i=1}^{l-1} b_i\right) \lambda_b^{(l-1)} + b_l \lambda_l}{\sum_{i=1}^{l-1} b_i + b_l} \\ &\leq \frac{\left(\sum_{i=1}^{l-1} b_i\right) \lambda_c^{(l-1)} + b \lambda_l}{\sum_{i=1}^{l-1} b_i + b_l} \end{aligned} \tag{5.45}$$

Since, $R_b^{l-1} \leq R_c^{l-1}$, and $\frac{\sum_{i=1}^{l-1} c_i}{\sum_{i=1}^{l-1} b_i} \leq \frac{c_l}{b_l}$, we have

$$\frac{\left(\sum_{i=1}^{l-1} b_i\right) \lambda_c^{(l-1)} + b \lambda_l}{\sum_{i=1}^{l-1} b_i + b_l} \leq \frac{\left(\sum_{i=1}^{l-1} c_i\right) \lambda_c^{(l-1)} + c \lambda_l}{\sum_{i=1}^{l-1} c_i + c_l}$$

$$= \frac{\sum_{i=1}^{l} c_i \lambda_i}{\sum_{i=1}^{l} c_i} \tag{5.46}$$

Hence, the Theorem 2 holds for all n.

5.5 Experiments

5.5.1 Datasets

In the experiments, we utilize three commonly-used HSI datasets to evaluate the performances of the methods under study. These datasets are the Indian Pines (IP), Salinas, and University of Houston 2013 (UH2013) datasets. The Indian Pines dataset has 200 spectral bands. The image size is 145 × 145, and it has 16 land-cover classes. The Salinas dataset consists of 204 spectral channels. Its size is 610 × 340, and it contains nine land-cover classes. Regarding the Houston 2013 dataset, the data has a size of 349 × 1905 and 144 channels. The image is labeled with 15 categories. The particulars of the three datasets employed in the experiment are shown in Table 5.2.

Table 5.2 The details of the datasets used for the evaluation of the investigated algorithms

NO	Indian pines		Salinas		UH2013	
	Landcover name	Pixels	Landcover name	Pixels	Landcover name	Pixels
1	Asphalt	46	Weed 1	2009	Healthy-grass	1251
2	Corn-notill	1428	Weed 2	3726	Stressed-grass	1254
3	Corn-mintill	830	Fallow	1976	Synthetic-grass	697
4	Corn	237	Fallow-plow	1394	Tress	1244
5	Grass-pasture	483	Fallow-smooth	2678	Soil	1242
6	Grass-trees	730	Stubble	3959	Water	325
7	Grass-pasture-mowed	28	Celery	3579	Residential	1268
8	Hay-windrowed	478	Grapes untrained	11,271	Commercial	1244
9	Oats	20	Soil	6203	Road	1252
10	Soybean-notill	972	Corn	3278	Highway	1227
11	Soybean-mintill	2455	Lettuce-4wk	1068	Railway	1235
12	Soybean-clean	593	Lettuce-5wk	1927	Parking-Lot 1	1233
13	Wheat	205	Lettuce-6wk	916	Parking-Lot 2	469
14	Woods	1265	Lettuce-7wk	1070	Tennis-Court	428
15	Buildings-grass-Trees-drives	386	Vineyard-untrained	7268	Running-Track	660
16	Stone-steel-towers	93	Vineyard-trellis	1807		

5.5.2 Baselines and Evaluation Metrics

To assess the clustering accuracy and real-time capabilities of the proposed L2GCC, we take into account 10 baseline methods for comparison. These include k-means [13], FCM [14], FCM-S1[17], spectral clustering (SC) [15], SSSC [22], S^5C [23], SGCNR [28], AE [43] + k-means, DEC [42], and CC [31]. Notably, k-means, FCM, FCM-S1, and SC are traditional clustering techniques devised for natural images. SC is a spectral clustering approach, while CC is a contrastive clustering method. SSSC and S5C fall under the category of sparse subspace clustering methods. Moreover, AE + k-means, DEC, and CC are deep clustering methods developed for large-scale HSI clustering. The hyperparameters of the above-mentioned methods are set as per their original papers.

In our experimental setup, five metrics are introduced for all the methods under study to evaluate their performances. These metrics are overall accuracy (OA), per-class accuracy (PA), kappa coefficient (κ), normalized mutual information (NMI), and adjusted rand index (ARI).

5.5.3 Experimental Settings

In our approach, there are principally six parameters that need to be set. These are the number of superpixels S (which are the graph nodes), the number of low-pass graph convolutional layers L, learning rate η, number of epochs T, number of initial centroids c, and distribution threshold δ. The optimal values of these parameters used in our proposed method are presented in Table 5.3. It must be emphasized that the value of δ is extremely small and, under normal conditions, will not be activated, except in the discrete scenario of clustering. The c initial centroids $\{\mu_j\}_{j=1}^{c}$ are derived through k-means clustering, and its value is equivalent to the number of land-covers present in the HSI. The dimensions of the three hidden layers are 168, 84, and 42 respectively.

The experiments in this chapter are carried out on an Intel i9-10900 K processor equipped with 3.70G of DDR4 RAM. For the graphic processing unit (GPU), an NVIDIA GeForce GTX 1080Ti having 11G of DDR4 RAM is utilized. In order to minimize random effects, we run all experiments ten times and present the average clustering performances, with Pytorch-Geometric serving as the back-end.

Table 5.3 Optimal values utilized in L2GCC

Dataset	S	L	T	η	c	δ (%)
IP	1000	3	200	0.001	16	0.1
Salinas	7000	3	200	0.001	16	0.1
UH 2013	14,000	3	200	0.001	15	0.1

5.5.4 Experimental Performances Comparison

In this part, the detailed quantitative clustering outcomes for the IP, Salinas, and UH2013 datasets are presented in Tables 5.5, and 5.6 respectively. The top-performing results are indicated in bold, while the second-best results are underlined. The associated visual clustering results are shown in Figs. 5.3, 5.4 and 5.5.

Quantitative results for the IP dataset: By looking at the quantitative clustering data in Table 5.4, several straightforward conclusions can be drawn. Firstly, L2GCC attains the most favorable outcomes across all crucial indicators in the experimental findings. This implies that our model has an excellent capacity to filter out interference noise. To be more specific, when compared to the second-best results, the outcomes of our proposed model show improvements of 18.37%, 16.37%, 8.72%, and 12.56% in OA, κ, NMI, and ARI respectively. Secondly, in contrast to classical methods such as k-means, FCM, and FCM-S1, scalable spectral/subspace clustering techniques can achieve better performances. This is because their mechanism is designed to assist with feature extraction. Specifically, SC, SSSC, and S^5C have higher clustering accuracies. The OAs of these three methods are enhanced by 3.42%, 0.17%, and 2.61% respectively when compared to k-means. Deep clustering algorithms (SGCNR, AE + k-means, DEC, CC, and L2GCC) are markedly superior to shallow methods (k-means, FCM, FCM-S1, SC). This is mainly due to the fact that deep learning can extract high-level features for clustering. In detail, compared to the best results among shallow methods, the clustering accuracies of deep clustering algorithms in terms of OA increase by 3.77%, 3.05%, 0.18%, and 13.16%. It is also worth noting that the graph-based clustering method SGCNR gets competitive results among deep clustering methods. This is because it can extract the complex nonlinear similarities among pixels by transforming high-dimensional spectral features into a graph-cut problem.

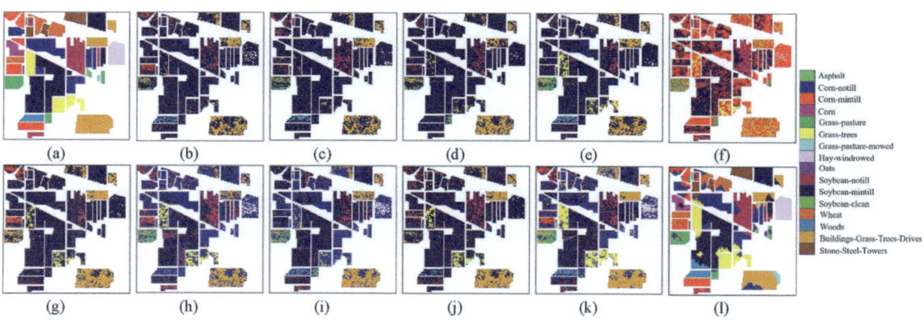

Fig. 5.3 The visual clustering map of investigated methods on IP dataset. **a** Ground-truth map; **b** k-means (OA = 38.11%); **c** FCM (OA = 37.57%); **d** FCM-S1(OA = 35.89%); **e** SC (OA = 41.53%); **f** SSSC (OA = 38.28%); **g** S^5C (OA = 40.72%); **h** SGCNR (OA = 45.30%); **i** AE + k-means (OA = 44.58%); **j** DEC (OA = 41.71%); **k** CC (OA = 55.14%); **l** L2GCC (OA = 73.51%)

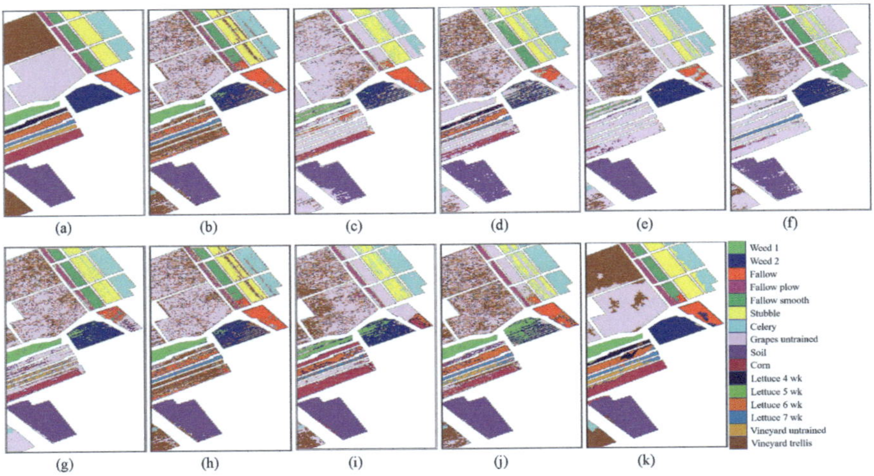

Fig. 5.4 The visual clustering map of investigated methods on Salinas dataset. **a** Ground-truth map; **b** k-means (OA = 67.99%); **c** FCM (OA = 56.73%); **d** FCM-S1(OA = 63.18%); **e** SSSC(OA = 52.43%); **f** S^5C(OA = 51.68%); **g** SGCNR (OA = 69.41%); **h** AE + k-means (OA = 65.68%); **i** DEC (OA = 62.57%); **j** CC (OA = 63.96%); **k** L2GCC (OA = 83.15%)

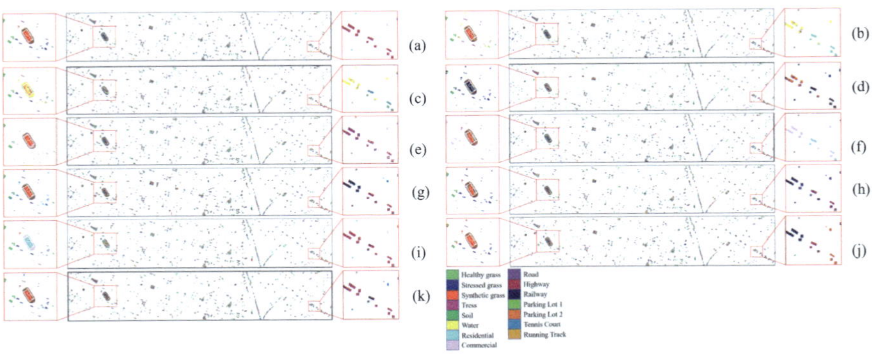

Fig. 5.5 The visual clustering map of investigated methods on UH2013 dataset. **a** Ground-truth map; **b** k-means (OA = 39.76%); **c** FCM (OA = 30.70%); **d** FCM-S1(OA = 31.82%); **e** SSSC(OA = 33.52%); **f** S^5C(OA = 31.67%); **g** SGCNR (OA = 44.62%); **h** AE + k-means (OA = 51.80%); **i** DEC (OA = 47.04%); **j** CC (OA = 53.48%); **k** L2GCC (OA = 64.12%)

Quantitative results for the Salinas dataset: From Table 5.5, the following conclusions can be drawn. First, among classical methods, k-means yields the best results, indicating that k-means can successfully distinguish more categories than the other two methods. Specifically, the OA of k-means is 38.11%, showing improvements of 0.54% and 2.22% compared to the values of FCM (37.57%) and FCM-S1 (35.89%) respectively. Second, in the case of spectral/subspace clustering methods, SSSC performs more effectively. Its OA (52.43%), κ (50.69%), NMI (64.23%), and ARI (46.76%) are enhanced by 0.75%, 0.34%, 0.96%, and 3.17% respectively compared

Table 5.4 Quantitative experimental performances of investigated methods on IP, bold denotes the best performances

No	*k*-means	FCM	FCM-S1	SC	SSSC	S^5C	SGCNR	AE + *k*-means	DEC	CC	L2GCC
1	0.0594	0.0567	0.0634	0.0000	0.0236	0.1125	0.0000	0.0870	0.0000	0.0870	**0.2543**
2	0.4563	0.5226	0.4426	0.0273	0.1836	0.2537	0.4398	0.1408	0.1877	0.2955	**0.6787**
3	0.1819	0.2118	0.1781	0.0048	0.3216	0.3576	0.0133	0.1940	0.2892	0.5795	**0.6028**
4	0.1237	0.1058	0.2109	0.0000	0.3018	0.1531	0.1477	0.1730	0.2405	0.8861	**0.9017**
5	0.3447	0.2946	0.3393	0.0166	0.6825	0.6279	0.4928	0.5217	0.0000	0.6584	**0.8236**
6	0.6901	0.7645	0.8008	0.0000	0.4913	0.5524	0.2123	0.9329	0.9726	0.9795	**1.0000**
7	0.0000	0.1043	0.0000	0.0000	0.6127	**0.7019**	0.0000	0.0000	0.0000	0.0000	0.0000
8	0.6239	0.8922	0.5706	**1.0000**	0.5736	0.5124	0.9582	0.7134	0.6464	**1.0000**	**1.0000**
9	0.0000	**0.6400**	0.0215	0.0000	0.0000	0.1329	0.1500	0.0000	0.0000	0.0000	0.3285
10	0.5654	0.2528	0.5268	0.0031	0.3162	0.2618	0.3735	0.5021	0.3693	0.4095	**0.7021**
11	0.4733	0.5141	0.5966	**0.9609**	0.3769	0.2235	0.6933	0.3752	0.3202	0.2957	0.6833
12	0.2592	0.2788	0.2553	0.0017	0.1823	0.0000	0.1754	0.1551	0.2749	**0.7437**	0.4564
13	0.3276	0.4289	0.2956	0.1463	0.6571	0.7531	0.9610	0.5024	0.3610	**1.0000**	**1.0000**
14	0.8559	0.8006	0.9173	**1.0000**	0.4839	0.4629	0.4877	0.7605	0.7763	0.6854	0.8346
15	0.2007	0.2869	0.2584	0.0000	0.2649	0.0000	0.1580	0.6995	0.7021	**1.0000**	**1.0000**
16	0.0000	0.0632	0.0000	0.7419	0.68310	0.7726	0.6882	0.5591	0.6022	0.0000	**0.8235**
OA	0.3811	0.3757	0.3589	0.4153	0.3828	0.4072	0.4530	0.4458	0.4171	0.5514	**0.7351**
κ	0.3572	0.2975	0.2782	0.2794	0.3326	0.3518	0.3730	0.3847	0.3591	0.5192	**0.6829**
NMI	0.4386	0.4380	0.4217	0.5041	0.4062	0.4317	0.4628	0.4527	0.4787	0.6644	**0.7516**
ARI	0.2195	0.2295	0.2070	0.2455	0.2138	0.2296	0.2571	0.2661	0.2968	0.4070	**0.5326**

Table 5.5 Quantitative experimental performances of investigated methods on Salinas, bold denotes the best performances. "oom" denotes out of memory

No	k-means	FCM	FCM-S1	SC	SSSC	S^5C	SGCNR	AE + k-means	DEC	CC	L2GCC
1	0.9985	0.4179	0.4860	OOM	0.0416	0.0000	0.0000	0.0000	0.9000	**1.0000**	**1.0000**
2	0.5698	0.5524	0.5637	OOM	0.9875	0.9628	0.6402	**1.0000**	0.7933	0.8969	0.9826
3	0.9741	0.8501	**1.0000**	OOM	0.0154	0.0434	0.3333	0.5501	0.0000	**1.0000**	0.9234
4	0.9865	0.0000	0.9537	OOM	0.8131	0.8512	**0.9950**	0.9340	0.5079	0.0000	0.8762
5	**0.7856**	0.5540	0.7365	OOM	0.8723	0.7526	0.6830	0.7367	0.7412	0.5310	0.7731
6	0.9952	0.9990	0.9704	OOM	0.9358	0.9832	0.9987	0.8406	0.8366	0.6603	**1.0000**
7	0.4810	0.0000	0.0003	OOM	0.5412	0.1126	**0.9798**	0.3328	0.6943	0.7499	0.7806
8	0.7309	0.7772	0.8412	OOM	0.4226	0.4917	0.5478	0.5008	**0.8565**	0.3615	0.8219
9	0.9750	0.6969	0.9602	OOM	0.5638	0.6826	0.7496	**0.9997**	0.9994	0.7201	0.9239
10	0.6169	0.5507	0.5429	OOM	0.1143	0.3158	0.8959	0.5863	0.3350	0.9451	**0.9137**
11	0.3370	0.0000	0.3013	OOM	0.6915	0.6213	0.0962	0.0000	0.0000	**1.0000**	0.7129
12	0.0273	0.0047	0.0000	OOM	0.4857	0.5184	0.8311	0.9460	0.8293	**0.9984**	0.9032
13	0.3548	0.8134	0.4613	OOM	0.0000	**0.9321**	0.0000	0.0000	0.0000	0.0000	0.6513
14	0.5584	0.6512	0.7469	OOM	0.1826	**0.8725**	0.6649	0.9645	0.0000	0.0000	0.6228
15	0.4994	0.4279	0.5064	OOM	0.4682	0.3948	0.0000	0.6237	0.0579	0.5687	**0.8027**
16	0.0000	0.8321	0.8433	OOM	0.9265	0.6617	0.8630	0.9917	0.9092	**1.0000**	0.8245
OA	0.6799	0.5673	0.6318	OOM	0.5243	0.5168	0.6941	0.6568	0.6257	0.6396	**0.8315**
κ	0.6572	0.5431	0.6202	OOM	0.5069	0.5035	0.7017	0.6206	0.5796	0.6123	**0.8226**
NMI	0.7356	0.6859	0.7089	OOM	0.6423	0.6327	0.7986	0.7720	0.7705	0.7806	**0.8569**
ARI	0.5466	0.4693	0.5119	OOM	0.4676	0.4359	0.5922	0.5548	0.5824	0.5330	**0.6926**

Table 5.6 Quantitative experimental performances of investigated methods on UH2013, bold denotes the best performances. "oom" denotes out of memory

No	*k*-means	FCM	FCM-S1	SC	SSSC	S^5C	SGCNR	AE + *k*-means	DEC	CC	LGCC
1	0.7926	0.4932	0.4762	OOM	0.5238	0.4813	0.4672	0.8129	0.8185	0.7506	**0.9017**
2	0.1436	0.2831	0.3017	OOM	0.3671	0.2516	0.3628	0.0973	**0.7783**	0.6938	0.4826
3	0.7638	0.0000	0.0000	OOM	0.0000	0.0000	0.6851	0.9842	0.4390	0.9900	**0.9999**
4	0.7024	0.3834	0.3921	OOM	0.4229	0.4420	0.6973	0.7436	0.0000	0.6624	**0.8731**
5	0.0000	0.6932	0.6273	OOM	0.2783	0.0000	0.0726	0.8285	**0.9815**	0.7198	0.7531
6	0.0000	0.0185	0.0372	OOM	0.1541	0.1266	0.1245	**0.7600**	0.0000	0.0000	0.6128
7	0.2416	0.0789	0.0564	OOM	0.0000	0.0510	0.3677	**0.8028**	0.0000	0.6088	0.6529
8	0.0000	0.0949	0.0629	OOM	0.2576	0.1932	0.1025	0.2291	0.2098	0.3778	**0.5326**
9	0.2671	0.1070	0.1324	OOM	0.0962	0.1224	0.3629	0.0000	**0.4744**	0.3011	0.0932
10	0.2935	0.2347	0.2179	OOM	0.2967	0.3125	0.2811	0.2771	**0.6544**	0.3325	0.5932
11	0.2613	**0.5417**	0.4386	OOM	0.3629	0.2718	0.3876	0.2777	0.0089	0.2874	0.4217
12	0.7132	0.8021	0.8211	OOM	0.7941	0.8530	0.6979	0.7875	0.5929	0.4039	**0.8871**
13	0.0000	0.0000	0.000	OOM	0.0000	0.0000	0.0000	0.0000	**0.6482**	0.6077	0.6168
14	**1.0000**	0.0000	0.0000	OOM	0.0000	0.0000	0.8143	0.9907	**1.0000**	0.0000	0.5132
15	0.3818	0.0000	0.0427	OOM	0.0000	0.0000	0.4537	0.5727	0.6258	0.9924	**1.0000**
OA	0.3976	0.3070	0.3182	OOM	0.3352	0.3167	0.4462	0.5180	0.4704	<u>0.5348</u>	**0.6412**
κ	0.3641	0.2456	0.2573	OOM	0.3219	0.3221	0.4315	0.4783	0.4278	<u>0.5008</u>	**0.6315**
NMI	0.5217	0.3623	0.3716	OOM	0.4153	0.4078	0.5521	0.5871	0.5660	<u>0.5949</u>	**0.6931**
ARI	0.2638	0.1488	0.1534	OOM	0.2035	0.1726	0.3029	0.3613	0.3330	<u>0.3977</u>	**0.5228**

to those of S^5C. Moreover, the performances of SSSC and S5C are better than those of classical methods. However, SC failed to complete the clustering due to out-of-memory issues, suggesting that SC needs improvement in its adaptability for clustering large datasets. Third, regarding the quantitative results of deep and shallow clustering methods, contrary to our expectations, deep clustering methods do not achieve the anticipated clustering advantages. This demonstrates that deep clustering methods are not always superior to shallow clustering methods. Nevertheless, SGCNR shows more competitive performance, with its OA improved by 3.73%, 6.84%, and 5.45% compared to the values of AE + k-means, DEC, and CC respectively. Fourth, the proposed L2GCC achieves the best clustering results. By comparing with the second-best method, it improves the OA, κ, NMI, and ARI by 13.74%, 12.09%, 5.84%, and 10.04% respectively, which validates the effectiveness of the proposed method.

Quantitative results for the UH2013 dataset: By analyzing the quantitative clustering data presented in Table 5.6, several conclusions can be readily drawn. First, when compared to the clustering outcomes of the IP and Salinas datasets, the results of all the investigated methods for the UH2013 dataset have significantly declined. The primary cause is that the UH2013 dataset is larger, featuring more pixels and intricate interconnections. This presents greater challenges to the algorithms under study, and SC experiences out-of-memory problems. Second, in contrast to the results for the Salinas dataset, deep clustering methods yield better results than shallow ones. This implies the strong adaptability of deep clustering methods for large-scale dataset clustering. They can measure the relationships between raw data by learning high-level semantic features. For instance, the OAs achieved by AE + k-means and CC are 51.80% and 53.48% respectively, which represent improvements of 12.04% and 13.72% over the best-performing shallow method. Additionally, compared to k-means, the deep-based AE + k-means shows a substantial enhancement in clustering accuracy. Third, L2GCC continues to achieve the best quantitative outcomes, further validating the superiority of our method's design. Overall, the proposed L2GCC method not only filters image noise effectively but also demonstrates good adaptability to various datasets.

Visual Clustering Results: The visual clustering maps of the investigated methods for the IP, Salinas, and UH2013 datasets are presented in Figs. 5.3, 5.4 and 5.5. From these results, it is straightforward to note that our LGCC generates the clustering maps with the fewest misclassifications, being remarkably nearer to the ground truth. Conversely, the comparison methods produce inferior clustering maps with distinct salt-and-pepper noises. This occurs since the low-pass graph filter utilized in the L2GCC is capable of retaining the low-frequency signal, which is beneficial for clustering. The layer-by-layer local features acquired by LGAT offer abundant features for clustering. Moreover, the high-level features learned by L2GCC assist in attaining a more precise clustering map.

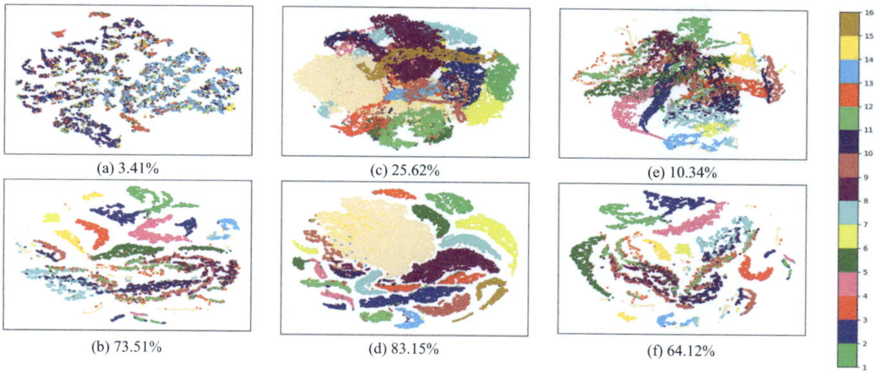

Fig. 5.6 2D visualization of the L2GCC on the IP (first column), Salinas (second column), and UH2013 (third column) at the epoch 0 and 200. Different colors in the maps denote different landcovers

5.5.5 T-SNE Data Distributions Visualization

In this experimental setup, the t-distributed stochastic neighbor embedding (t-SNE) [44] is employed to visualize how the data distributions of the IP, Salinas, and UH2013 datasets change during the training of L2GCC. Figure 5.6 shows the 2D visualizations of L2GCC on these three datasets at epoch 0 and 200. From the outcomes, it can be deduced that as the training iteration of our L2GCC increases, it is able to clearly differentiate between different types of nodes. Specifically, in the original three datasets (first row), there were small inter-class dissimilarities and large intra-class variations. With network training, L2GCC has the ability to learn highly discriminative feature representations. These representations are not only compact within classes but also well-separated between classes, thereby contributing to a higher clustering accuracy.

5.5.6 Parameter Study

In this part, we explore the impact of the number of superpixels S (which are graph nodes), the number of low-pass graph convolutional layers L, the learning rate η, and the number of epochs T on the performance of L2GCC. We group these four parameters into two sets and use a grid search strategy to determine the optimal settings. The experimental set-ups are the same as those in Sect. 5.3, and the clustering accuracy OA is used to report the performance of our L2GCC method with different parameter configurations. The parameter-sensitivity results of the two groups of parameters for IP, Salinas, and UH2013 are presented in Figs. 5.7 and 5.8.

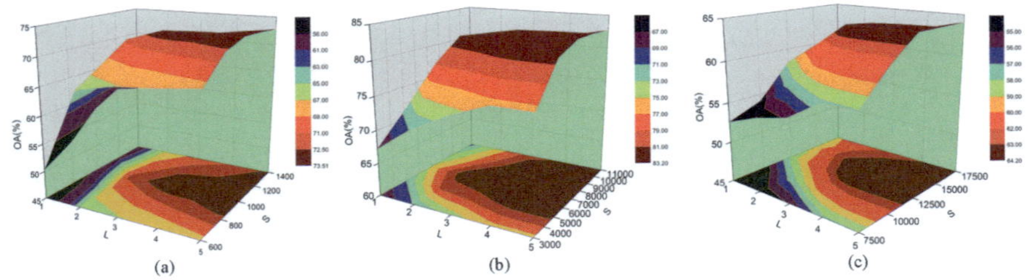

Fig. 5.7 3D visualization of the LGCC with different S and L on the Indian pines (**a**), Salinas (**b**), and UH2013 (**c**) datasets

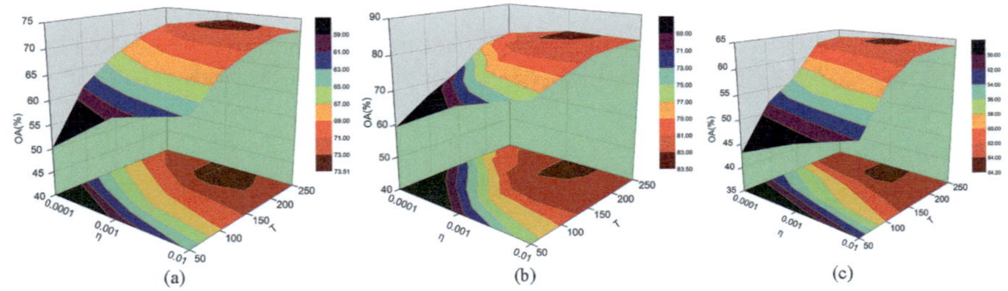

Fig. 5.8 3D visualization of LGCC with different T and η on the Indian Pines (**a**), Salinas (**b**), and UH2013 (**c**) datasets

***S* and *L* effect analysis**: The parameter-sensitivity results of S and L on L2GCC a re shown in Fig. 5.7. In the experiment, on the IP dataset, S varies from 600 to 1400 with an increment of 250. On the Salinas dataset, it ranges from 3000 to 11,000 with an interval of 2000, and on the UH2013 dataset, from 7500 to 17,500. The value of L is set from 1 to 5. Additionally, we keep T and η fixed as shown in Table 5.3. From the results, the OAs on the three datasets improve as S increases. Nevertheless, the clustering accuracy stops rising once S reaches a certain threshold. A larger S implies smaller superpixels, enabling us to retain more local spatial features of HSI for clustering. However, a larger S also results in more graph nodes, and an excessive number of graph nodes poses challenges to network feature exraction and escalates the computational complexity. As a result, for the IP, Salinas, and UH2013 datasets, S is set to 1000, 7000, and 14,000 respectively. Regarding L, a bigger L can efficiently learn the high-level features of graphs. But it requires more weight parameters and more time for network training. In our L2GCC, we find that the optimal value of L is 3 on three datasets.

***T* and η effect analysis**: In the experimental procedure, we alter T from 50 to 250 with a step size of 50, and η is set at values of 0.0001, 0.001, and 0.01. Additionally, S, L, m, and δ are held constant as per Table 5.3. The parameter-sensitivity outcomes of T and η on L2GCC are shown in Fig. 5.8. A large η allows for quicker training of the network parameters. However, it often fails to yield an optimal solution, and the final results tend to be unstable. Thus, in our L2GCC approach, η is set to 0.001. It is also important to note that T is strongly associated with η, and a bigger T implies that more time is required for network training. From the experimental results, we can see that the optimal results are achieved when T is 200.

5.5.7 *Ablation Study*

In this experiment, we evaluate the contributions of the pixel to region transformation module (PRT), Low-pass GCN, and LGAT within L2GCC in enhancing the HSI clustering for the IP, Salinas, and UH2013 datasets. The experimental configuration remains the same as that in Sect. 5.5.3. The OA is used to report the clustering accuracy, and the findings are presented in Table 5.7. For the sake of simplicity, we use "L2GCC-v_1"- "L2GCC-v_7" to represent the reduced methods. From the results, it is evident that L2GCC attains the best performances. Specifically, the clustering accuracies of LGCC-v_2 are better than the values of L2GCC-v_1, and L2GCC-v_7 performs better than L2GCC-v_3, which indicates that PRT can improve the clustering accuracy. Compared with LGCC-v_1, L2GCC-v_3 achieves a superior result, and LGCC-v_5 outperforms LGGCC-v_4, which verifies Low-pass GCN plays an important role in the proposed methods. Similarly, we can observe that the OA of L2GCC-v_3 is higher than L2GCC-v_1, and L2GCC-v_6 achieves a superior result to that of L2GCC-v_2, which shows the superiority of LGAT. Thus, PRT, Low-pass GCN, and LGAT all contribute to the improvement of the clustering accuracy in our L2GCC.

5.6 Conclusion

In this chapter, a new self-supervised L2GCC framework has been devised to enhance the clustering performance for large-scale HSI datasets. In particular, a region transformation module has been created. Its function is to transform the local spatial-spectral features of the HSI, thereby reducing the computational complexity. A locality-preserving low-pass graph convolutional embedding autoencoder has been developed. This autoencoder can efficiently learn high-level hidden representations at the superpixel level. In it, the low-pass GCN is designed to extract smoother features, while the layer-wise GAT is designed to extract locality features. Additionally, the Kullback–Leibler (KL) Divergence is employed to assess the graph reconstruction loss. Self-training clustering is carried out using soft labels generated from the graph embedding. The L2GCC algorithm combines the locality-preserving low-pass graph convolutional embedding autoencoder and self-training clustering. These two components are mutually advantageous. When compared with state-of-the-art clustering methods, L2GCC demonstrates excellent model design and superiority. The clustering accuracy OAs on IP, Salinas, and UH2013 are 73.51%, 83.15%, and 64.12% respectively.

Table 5.7 Ablation study results on IP, Salinas, UH2013. The OA indexes (%) is reported. The pixel to region transformation module (HSI pre-processing) is simplified as "PRT"

Name		L2GCC-v_1	L2GCC-v_2	L2GCC-v_3	L2GCC-v_4	L2GCC-v_5	L2GCC-v_6	L2GCC-v_7	L2GCC
Module	PRT	–	✓	–	–	–	✓	✓	✓
	Low-pass GCN	–	–	✓	–	✓	–	✓	✓
	LGAT	–	–	–	✓	✓	✓	–	✓
Dataset	IP	59.76	65.23	64.26	63.28	66.82	69.35	72.39	**73.51**
	Salinas	66.38	72.34	71.72	70.61	73.39	78.23	82.26	**83.15**
	UH2013	54.19	59.73	59.81	53.33	55.17	58.76	62.75	**64.12**

In comparison to supervised and semi-supervised methods, unsupervised methods need improvement in terms of clustering accuracy, especially for large-scale HSIs. Nevertheless, the success of L2GCC indicates the broad potential of unsupervised clustering methods in HSI classification. In future, efforts will be made to improve the HSI pre-processing method and to explore more forms of GCN-based self-supervised autoencoders, such as GCN-GAN, among others.

References

1. Rasti B et al (2020) Feature extraction for hyperspectral imagery: the evolution from shallow to deep: overview and toolbox. IEEE Geosci Remote Sens Mag 8(4):60–88 (2020) https://doi.org/10.1109/MGRS.2020.2979764
2. Chen Y, Xiao X, Peng C, Lu G, Zhou Y (2022) Low-rank tensor graph learning for multi-view subspace clustering. IEEE Trans Circ Syst Video Technol 32(1):92–104
3. Ding Y, Zhao X, Zhang Z, Cai W, Yang N (2022) Graph sample and aggregate-attention network for hyperspectral image classification. IEEE Geosci Rem Sens Lett 19:1–5, Art no. 5504205, https://doi.org/10.1109/LGRS.2021.3062944
4. Ding Y, Zhao X, Zhang Z, Cai W, Yang N (2021) Multiscale graph sample and aggregate network with context-aware learning for hyperspectral image classification. IEEE J Select Top Appl Earth Observ Rem Sens 14:4561–4572 (2021) https://doi.org/10.1109/JSTARS.2021.3074469
5. Ding Y, Zhao X, Zhang Z, Cai W, Yang N, Zhan Y (2022) Semi-supervised locality preserving dense graph neural network with ARMA filters and context-aware learning for hyperspectral image classification. IEEE Trans Geosci Remote Sens 60:1–12, Art no. 5511812. https://doi.org/10.1109/TGRS.2021.3100578
6. Peng Z, Jia Y, Liu H, Hou J, Zhang Q (2022) Maximum entropy subspace clustering network. IEEE Trans Circ Syst Video Technol 32:2199–2210
7. Cai Y, Zhang Z, Yan Q, Zhang D, Banu MJ (2021) Densely connected convolutional extreme learning machine for hyperspectral image classification. Neurocomputing 434:21–32
8. Ding Y, Zhang Z, Zhao X, Cai W, He F, Cai Y (2022) Deep hybrid: multi-graph neural network collaboration for hyperspectral image classification. Defence Technol. https://doi.org/10.1016/j.dt.2022.02.007
9. Cai Y, Zhang Z, Cai Z, Liu X, Jiang X, Yan Q (2021) Graph convolutional subspace clustering: a robust subspace clustering framework for hyperspectral image. IEEE Trans Geosci Remote Sens 59(5):4191–4202
10. Vidal R (2011) Subspace clustering. IEEE Signal Process Mag 28(2):52–68
11. Lei J, Li X, Peng B, Fang L, Ling N, Huang Q (2021) Deep spatialspectral subspace clustering for hyperspectral image. IEEE Trans Circuits Syst Video Technol 31(7):2686–2697
12. Peng X, Feng J, Zhou JT, Lei Y, Yan S (2020) Deep subspace clustering. IEEE Trans Neural Netw Learn Syst 31(12):5509–5521
13. Kanungo T, Mount DM, Netanyahu NS, Piatko CD, Silverman R, Wu AY (2002) An efficient k-means clustering algorithm: analysis and implementation. IEEE Trans Pattern Anal Mach Intell 24(7):881–892
14. Ng AY, Jordan MI, Weiss Y (2002) On spectral clustering: analysis and an algorithm. Proc Adv Neural Inf Process Syst (NIPS) 849–856
15. Yang T, Lee C, Yen S (2009) Fuzzy objective functions for robust pattern recognition. In: 2009 IEEE international conference on fuzzy systems, pp 2057–2062
16. Shah CA, Arora MK, Varshney PK (2004) Unsupervised classification of hyperspectral data: an ICA mixture model-based approach. Int J Remote Sens 25(2):481–487

17. Chen S, Zhang D (2004) Robust image segmentation using FCM with spatial constraints based on new kernel-induced distance measure. IEEE Trans Syst Man Cybern Part B (Cybern) 34(4):1907–1916
18. Liu H, Jia Y, Hou J, Zhang Q (2022) Global-local balanced low-rank approximation of hyperspectral images for classification. IEEE Trans Circ Syst Video Technol 32(4):2013–2024
19. Lin J, He C, Wang ZJ, Li S (2017) Structure preserving transfer learning for unsupervised hyperspectral image classification. IEEE Geosci Rem Sens Lett 14(10):1656–1660
20. Murphy JM, Maggioni M (2019) Unsupervised clustering and active learning of hyperspectral images with nonlinear diffusion. IEEE Trans Geosci Remote Sens 57(3):1829–1845
21. Elhamifar E, Vidal R (2013) Sparse subspace clustering: algorithm, theory, and applications. IEEE Trans Pattern Anal Mach Intell 35(11):2765–2781
22. Peng X, Tang H, Zhang L, Yi Z, Xiao S (2016) A unified framework for representation-based subspace clustering of out-of-sample and largescale data. IEEE Trans Neural Netw Learn Syst 27(12):2499–2512
23. Matsushima S, Brbic M (2019) Selective sampling-based scalable sparse subspace clustering. In: Wallach H, Larochelle H, Beygelzimer A, d'Alche-Buc F, Fox E, Garnett R (eds) Advances in neural information processing systems. Curran Associates, Inc., vol 32
24. Ding Y, Zhang Z, Zhao X, Hong D, Li W, Cai W, Zhan Y (2022) AF2GNN: graph convolution with adaptive filters and aggregator fusion for hyperspectral image classification. Inf Sci 602:201–219
25. Fan J, Chen T, Lu S (2018) Superpixel guided deep-sparse-representation learning for hyperspectral image classification. IEEE Trans Circ Syst Video Technol 28(11):3163-3173
26. Xie J, Girshick R, Farhadi A (2016) Unsupervised deep embedding for clustering analysis. In: Balcan MF, Weinberger KQ (eds) Proceedings of the 33rd international conference on machine learning. Proceedings of machine learning research. PMLR, New York, USA, vol 48, pp 478–487
27. Cai Y, Zeng M, Cai Z, Liu X, Zhang Z (2021) Graph regularized residual subspace clustering network for hyperspectral image clustering. Inf Sci 578:85–101
28. Wang R, Nie F, Wang Z, He F, Li X (2019) Scalable graph-based clustering with nonnegative relaxation for large hyperspectral image. IEEE Trans Geosci Remote Sens 57(10):7352–7364
29. Lei J, Li X, Peng B, Fang L, Ling N, Huang Q (2021) Deep spatial-spectral subspace clustering for hyperspectral image. IEEE Trans Circ Syst Video Technol 31(7):2686–2697
30. Hou S, Shi H, Cao X, Zhang X, Jiao L (2021) Hyperspectral imagery classification based on contrastive learning. IEEE Trans Geosci Remote Sens 60:1–13
31. Li Y, Hu P, Liu Z, Peng D, Zhou JT, Peng X (2021) Contrastive clustering. In: 2021 AAAI conference on artificial intelligence (AAAI) 35(10):8547–8555
32. Bruna J, Zaremba W, Szlam A, Le Cun Y (2013) Spectral networks and locally connected networks on graphs, arXiv preprintarXiv:1312.6203
33. Kipf T, Welling M (2016) Variational graph auto-encoders. arXiv preprintarXiv:1611.07308
34. Wang C, Pan S, Long G, Zhu X, Jing J (2017) Mgae: marginalized graph autoencoder for graph clustering. ACM
35. Park J, Lee M, Chang HJ, Lee K, Choi J (2019) Symmetric graph convolutional autoencoder for unsupervised graph representation learning. In: Proceedings of the IEEE international conference on computer vision, pp 6519–6528
36. Zhang X, Liu H, Li Q, Wu X (2019) Attributed graph clustering via adaptive graph convolution. In: Proceedings of the 28th international joint conference on artificial intelligence. AAAI Press, pp 4327–4333
37. Pan S, Hu R, Long G, Jiang J, Yao L, Zhang C (2018) Adversarially regularized graph autoencoder for graph embedding. IJCAI 2609–2615
38. Horn R, Johnson C (2012) Matrix analysis. Cambridge University Press
39. Xie J, Girshick R, Farhadi A (2016) Unsupervised deep embedding for clustering analysis. ICML, PMLR, New York, pp 478–487
40. Scholkopf B, Smola A, Muller K-R (1998) Nonlinear component analysis as a kernel eigenvalue problem. Neural Comput 10(5):1299–1319

41. Achanta R, Shaji A, Smith K, Lucchi A, Fua P, Strunk S (2012) SLIC superpixels compared to state-of-the-art superpixel methods. IEEE Trans Pattern Anal Mach Intell 34(11):2274–2282
42. Xie J, Girshick R, Farhadi A (2016) Unsupervised deep embedding for clustering analysis. In: Balcan MF, Weinberger KQ (eds)Proceedings of the 33rd international conference on machine learning, ser. Proceedings of machine learning research. PMLR, New York, pp 478–487
43. Hinton GE, Salakhutdinov RR (2006) Reducing the dimensionality of data with neural networks. Science 313(5786):504–507
44. Van der Maaten L, Hinton G (2008) Visualizing data using t-SNE. J Mach Learn Res 9(11)

Chapter 6
Adaptive Homophily Clustering for Hyperspectral Image

6.1 Introduction

Hyperspectral image (HSI) has the distinct advantage of obtaining continuous spectral details about target objects. Due to this, it has found extensive applications across a wide range of fields [1, 2]. These include earth observation [3], environmental monitoring [4], military detection [5], and resource exploration [6]. HSI is replete with potential for feature identification and classification, making HSI interpretation a subject of substantial research importance. Nevertheless, HSIs come with high dimensionality, substantial redundancy, and high computational complexity. These characteristics pose significant hurdles in their analysis, processing, and interpretation [7, 8]. Conventionally, a large number of labeled samples are typically utilized to train interpretation methods for HSI interpretation. This approach is not only costly but also labor-intensive and time-consuming [9, 10]. Consequently, the study of unsupervised hyperspectral image classification methods for land-cover classification analysis is highly significant. Clustering analysis, an unsupervised learning approach, can group similar pixels in HSI into separate clusters. This enables the extraction of valuable information without the need for pre-labeled training samples, offering a potential solution to surmount the aforementioned challenges [11, 12].

Previously, several clustering methods originally created for natural images have been applied to HSI. These include K-means clustering [13], possibilistic C-means (PCM) [14], spectral clustering [15], fuzzy C-means [16], and density peak clustering [17]. Although these methods have had some achievements in HSI clustering, they solely make use of prototypical features that carry a large amount of redundant information. As a result, they encounter difficulties in effective dimension reduction, noise management, and algorithm optimization [18]. Due to these limitations, the clustering accuracy is not satisfactory, and their wide-scale application has been constrained. Subsequently, in order to deal with the interference of redundant information, some subspace clustering (SC) algorithms [9] were devised. These algorithms map high-dimensional image information into a low-dimensional information space. Examples

Y. Ding et al., *Graph Neural Network for Hyperspectral Image Clustering*, Intelligent Perception and Information Processing, https://doi.org/10.1007/978-981-96-7710-8_6

are parse subspace clustering (SSC) [19], nonnegative matrix factorization (NMF) [20], and low-rank representation (LRR) [21]. However, these methods only concentrate on extracting spectral features and overlook the intrinsic relationship of spatially identifiable features [22]. To make more flexible use of spatial-spectral information, Zhang et al. [23] employed a fuzzy similarity measure to determine the boundaries of different categories. Zhai et al. [24] further enhanced the effective utilization of spatial information by adding an ℓ_2-norm regularization based on SSC. Inspired by graph learning for extracting potential relationships between nodes, some graph subspace clustering algorithms were developed. For instance, Wang et al. [25] proposed a scalable graph-based clustering (SGCNR), in which the computational complexity is decreased through nonnegative relaxation. Nevertheless, the traditional clustering methods mentioned above are shallow classifiers based on original features and often rely on hand-crafted spectral-spatial features. These features are frequently incapable of extracting representative features [26]. These drawbacks make it challenging to explore deep semantic information and adapt to the spectral variations of HSI.

Motivated by the progress in deep clustering learning, numerous deep clustering techniques have been utilized to surmount the limitations of traditional clustering approaches. In these methods, hyper-parameters are adjusted via self-supervised training, and discriminative spatial-spectral features are learned for clustering purposes. Generally, most deep clustering methods can be categorized into three components: a deep feature extractor, a representative feature expressor, and a self-training optimizer. For instance, Zhang et al. [27] constructed spatial-spectral similarity graphs based on superpixels. A dual graph autoencoder was then employed to concurrently extract and decode the spatial-spectral features. Cai et al. [18] put forward a contrastive subspace clustering method called NCSC. In this method, a pooling autoencoder was developed to learn the superpixel-level latent subspace and its representation. These methods have made substantial efforts to apply deep clustering in HSI clustering. However, they often struggle to more effectively capture complex spatial structural information, which leads to less-than-optimal clustering performances.

Lately, the evolution of graph clustering methods has enabled deep clustering techniques to efficiently encode spatial structural information. This has shifted deep clustering methods from solely handling Euclidean data to dealing with non-Euclidean geometric graph-structured data. A multitude of structural graph clustering networks have been created, and they have shown outstanding efficacy in learning structural information via graph embeddings. For example, in the work of [28], a low-pass graph filter was devised to learn smoother structural features, thereby enhancing the clustering accuracy. Luo et al. [29] designed a dual transformer-based autoencoder to extract long-dependency graph features, which precisely represented the graph structure features. In an attempt to explore target-oriented graph clustering methods, in [30] the graph attention network (GAT) was used to aggregate the correlation information of neighboring nodes, and the development of self-training modules led to better clustering performance. Simultaneously, to extract higher-order and global structural correlations, several high-order graphs such as the pixel-superpixel graph [31], multiview graph, and hypergraph [32] have come into existence to capture the structure as well as spectral-spatial information. Despite the significant headway made in graph-based clustering methods for HSI, the filters in current graph networks are inflexible. They lack sufficient capacity to process signal features for diverse nodes, which results in subpar clustering accuracy for large-scale HSI [33]. Additionally, mainstream graph networks generally do not permit the modification of the original graph according to different clustering tasks. Instead, the graph remains static and unaltered during network training. This constraint makes it arduous to correct incorrect edge connections in the original graph, severely impeding the improvement of HIS clustering accuracy, particularly in large graphs.

To tackle these issues, we put forward a new technique named Adaptive Homophily Structure Graph Clustering (AHSGC) for HSIs. Initially, our method utilizes a superpixel segmentation approach to create the graph structure. Then, we engineer a graph convolution encoder that comes with an adaptive filter. This filter has the capacity to dynamically capture both the high- and low- frequency features of the graph. Furthermore, we develop a graph embedding clustering self-training decoder to obtain appropriate graph representations. We also introduce a structure homophily-enhanced learning mechanism. This mechanism uses orient correlation estimation to evaluate pairwise correlations between nodes via a hierarchical correlation estimation framework. It is accompanied by intra-cluster edge recovery and inter-cluster edge removal mechanisms, enabling the graph structure to be adjusted dynamically according to particular clustering tasks. Subsequently, we carry out joint network optimization. We use a self-training loss and a graph reconstruction loss to promote graph self-training and updates. Finally, we apply K-means clustering to represent the latent features. The advantage of the proposed sub-network is its capability to adaptively optimize the graph structure in accordance with the clustering tasks. This, in turn, improves the accuracy and robustness of HSI clustering. By making dynamic adjustments to the graph based on the learned correlations and features, our method can more effectively capture the underlying relationships in the data, resulting in enhanced clustering results.

The novel contributions of our AHSGC are presented as follows:

(1) We introduce a graph convolution encoder featuring an adaptive filter. This filter enables the adaptive extraction of both high-frequency and low-frequency elements on the graph.
(2) We create a homophily-enhanced structure learning approach. This approach allows for the dynamic modification of the graph structure in line with diverse clustering tasks, through the removal of inter-cluster edges and the recovery of intra-cluster edges.
(3) We make use of an auxiliary distribution to carry out self-training for AHSGC. Subsequently, k-means is employed to perform the clustering process.

6.2 Related Work

6.2.1 Graph and Graph Filter

(1) Graph Definition

Consider an undirected graph $\mathcal{G} = (\mathcal{V}, \mathcal{E}, \boldsymbol{A})$ which has N nodes, C classes and edge set $\mathcal{E}$, where $\mathcal{V} = \{v_1, v_2, \ldots, v_N\}$, $\boldsymbol{X} \in \mathbb{R}^{N\times D}$ and $\boldsymbol{A} \in \mathbb{R}^{N\times N}$ are the feature matrix and adjacency matrix of the constructed graph, respectively.

The relevant notations are summarized in Table 6.1.

(2) Graph Filter Definiti

For a discrete input signal $\hat{f}_{\text{in}}$ (ξ pon performing the Fourier convolution operation as described in [34], the resulting output signal in the time-domain $f_{\text{out}}(t)$ can be expressed as

$$f_{\text{out}}(t) = \int_{-\infty}^{+\infty} \hat{f}_{\text{in}}(\xi)\hat{h}(\xi)\mathrm{e}^{2\pi i\xi t}d\xi = \int_{-\infty}^{+\infty} f_{\text{in}}(\tau)h(t-\tau)d\tau = (f_{\text{in}} * h)(t) \quad (6.1)$$

Table 6.1 Main notions summary

Notation	Meaning
$rm\mathcal{G} = (\mathcal{V}, \mathcal{E}, \boldsymbol{A})$	Graph $\mathcal{G}$ with edge $\mathcal{E}$ and node V
N	Graph node number
$\boldsymbol{X} \in \mathbb{R}^{N\times D}$	Node feature matrix
$\boldsymbol{X}_i$	i-th node feature
$\boldsymbol{A} \in \mathbb{R}^{N\times N}$	Adjacency matrix
S_i	The i th superpixel
n_i	The number of pixels contained in S_i
$\boldsymbol{Z} \in \mathbb{R}^{hw\times N}$	The correlation matrix
h, w, and b	The height, width, and number of bands of the HSI
$\boldsymbol{S} \in \mathbb{R}^{N\times N}$	Node similarity matrix
$\boldsymbol{H}$	Graph Laplacian filter
$\boldsymbol{F}_{\text{A}}$	Adaptive graph filter
$\boldsymbol{A}_{rw}$	Randomly wandering normalized affine matrix
$\boldsymbol{Z}_i$ and $\boldsymbol{Z}$	The i-th layer and graph encoder output
$\boldsymbol{Z} \in \mathbb{R}^{N\times D}$	The clustering-oriented node features
ξ	Intra-cluster edge recovery ratio
η	Inter-cluster edge removal ratio
γ	High-confidence node extraction ratio
$\mathcal{L}_c$, $\mathcal{L}_g$	Self-training loss and graph reconstruction loss

where the unit of ξ is Hz, and $\hat{h}(\xi)$ is a frequency response function.

Based on Eq. (6.1), the graph convolution operation with respect to the discrete graph node signal $\hat{h}(\lambda_k)$ can be defined in the following way

$$f_{\text{out}}(i)=\sum_{k=1}^{n}\hat{f}_{\text{in}}(\lambda_k)\hat{h}(\lambda_k)\boldsymbol{v}_k(i) \tag{6.2}$$

where $\hat{f}_{\text{in}}(\lambda_k)$ denotes the magnitude of the graph signal at the frequency λ_k, $\boldsymbol{v}_k(\cdot)$ is the Fourier basis of the graph signal, and i stands for the i th element of $\boldsymbol{v}_k(\cdot)$. In Eq. (6.2), the integral operation present in Eq. (6.1) is substituted by a summation operation.

If we set $\hat{f}_{in}=U^T f_{in}$, then we are able to simplify Eq. (6.2) to matrix form as

$$\begin{aligned}
f_{\text{out}}&=\sum_{k=1}^{n}h(\lambda_k)\hat{f}_{\text{in}}(\lambda_k)\boldsymbol{v}_k=\begin{bmatrix} | & | & \dots & | \\ \boldsymbol{v}_1 & \boldsymbol{v}_2 & \dots & \boldsymbol{v}_n \\ | & | & \dots & | \end{bmatrix}\begin{bmatrix} h(\lambda_1)\hat{f}_{in}(\lambda_1) \\ h(\lambda_2)\hat{f}_{in}(\lambda_2) \\ \dots \\ h(\lambda_n)\hat{f}_{\text{in}}(\lambda_n) \end{bmatrix} \\
&=\begin{bmatrix} | & | & \dots & | \\ \boldsymbol{v}_1 & \boldsymbol{v}_2 & \dots & \boldsymbol{v}_n \\ | & | & \dots & | \end{bmatrix}\begin{bmatrix} h(\lambda_1) & \dots & 0 \\ \vdots & \ddots & \vdots \\ 0 & \dots & h(\lambda_n) \end{bmatrix}\begin{bmatrix} - & \boldsymbol{v}_1^T & - \\ - & \boldsymbol{v}_2^T & - \\ - & \dots & - \\ - & \boldsymbol{v}_n^T & - \end{bmatrix} f_{in} \\
&=\boldsymbol{U}\begin{bmatrix} h(\lambda_1) & \dots & 0 \\ \vdots & \ddots & \vdots \\ 0 & \dots & h(\lambda_n) \end{bmatrix}\boldsymbol{U}^T f_{\text{in}}=\boldsymbol{U}\boldsymbol{\Lambda}_h\boldsymbol{U}^T f_{in}=\mathbf{H}f_{\text{in}}
\end{aligned} \tag{6.3}$$

Accordingly, the graph filter can be defined as

$$\boldsymbol{H}=\boldsymbol{U}\boldsymbol{\Lambda}_h\boldsymbol{U}^T\in\mathbb{R}^{n\times n},\boldsymbol{H}:\mathbb{R}^n\to\mathbb{R}^n \tag{6.4}$$

where $\boldsymbol{\Lambda}_{\text{h}}$ serves as the frequency response matrix associated with the graph filter.

6.2.2 Homophily-Enhanced Graph Learning

For a given graph having $\mathcal{G}=\{\boldsymbol{X},\boldsymbol{A}\}$ with C classes, if we designate the node $\boldsymbol{v}_i$ as y_i, the concept of edge homogeneity, which represents the proportion of edges that connect nodes within the same class to the overall number of edges in the graph, can be defined as

$$h(\mathcal{G}, \{\mathrm{y_i}; \mathrm{v_i} \in \mathcal{V}\}) = \frac{1}{|\mathcal{E}|} \sum_{(v_i, v_j) \in \mathcal{E}} \mathbb{I}(\mathrm{y_i} = \mathrm{y_j}) \tag{6.5}$$

where $\mathbb{I}(\cdot)$ is an indicator function

The objective of graph clustering is to partition the node set $\mathcal{V}$ into class C. In other words, it involves allocating each node $\boldsymbol{v}_i$ to a particular cluster based on its unique features, and this can be represented as

$$\begin{cases} \min \sum_{i=1}^{m} \sum_{j=1}^{m} d(i, j) = \min \sum_{i=1}^{m} \sum_{j=1}^{m} f(\boldsymbol{x}_i) - f(\boldsymbol{x}_j)_2^2 \\ \max \sum_{\alpha=1}^{c} \sum_{\beta=1}^{c} d(\alpha, \beta) = \max \sum_{\alpha=1}^{c} \sum_{\beta=1}^{c} y(\boldsymbol{c}_\alpha) - y(\boldsymbol{c}_\beta)_2^2 \end{cases} \tag{6.6}$$

where $f(\cdot)$ is a function utilized for mapping the optimal spatial-spectral data of a node, while $y(\cdot)$ is a function applied to compute the characteristics of a cluster. The variable m represents the count of nodes within a particular cluster.

6.3 Proposed Method

In this part, the overall architecture of AHSGC is initially expounded. Subsequently, the aspects of HSI Preprocessing and Initial Graph Construction are presented. Finally, the structural particulars of AHSGC, namely the Adaptive Filter Graph Encoder, Graph Embedding Clustering Self-Training Decoder, Homophily-enhanced Structure Learning, and Joint Network Optimization, are comprehensively described.

6.3.1 Overall AHSGC Framework

The AHSGC we proposed is principally composed of five components. These are the Adaptive Filter Graph Encoder, the Graph Embedding Clustering Self-Training Decoder, the Homophily-enhanced Structure Learning, the Joint Network Optimization, and the HSI Preprocessing and Initial Graph Construction module. The overall framework of AHSGC is depicted in Fig. 6.1. The primary functions of these five components are as follows

- **HSI Preprocessing and Initial Graph Construction:** We implement a superpixel segmentation approach. This method transforms HSIs from pixels to regions. It has the advantage of maintaining local spatial-spectral structure information and simultaneously reducing the number of nodes.
- **Adaptive Filter Graph Encoder:** The input to AHSGC is the superpixel-level graph. To extract and filter both low- and high- frequency features on the graph

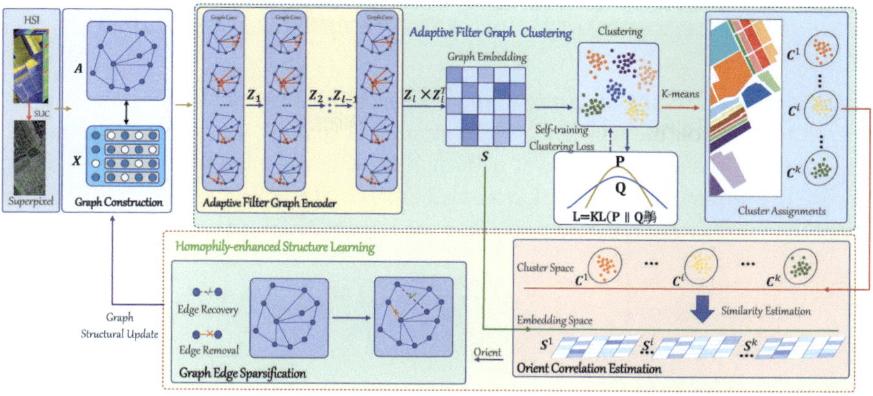

Fig. 6.1 Overview of AHSGC for HSI. AHSGC is primarily composed of five components: HSI Preprocessing and initial graph construction, an adaptive filter graph encoder, a graph embedding clustering self-training decoder, homophily-enhanced structure learning, and a joint network optimization module. The HSI Preprocessing and initial graph construction are introduced to convert the pixels in HSI into regions that preserve locality and build the original graph. An adaptive filter graph encoder is created to extract and filter the low-and high-frequency features on the graph. The graph embedding clustering self-training decoder is employed to perform self-training and decode the extracted features. The homophily-enhanced structure learning is developed to modify the graph based on the clustering task. The joint network optimization module is put forward to improve the structural consistency and graph edge sparsification of the graph and train the proposed network

for clustering purposes, we design an adaptive graph filter. This is achieved by aggregating neighbor information using the adaptive graph filter.

- **Graph Embedding Clustering Self-Training Decoder:** We use an auxiliary distribution to carry out self-training for AHSGC. Subsequently, k-means is employed to perform the clustering process.
- **Homophily-enhanced Structure Learning:** In order to get sparser edges, we have developed mechanisms for removing inter-cluster edges and recovering intra-cluster edges. These mechanisms enable the graph structure to be adjusted dynamically in accordance with various clustering tasks.
- **Joint Network Optimization:** We put forward a new joint objective loss. This loss aims to improve the structural consistency and graph edge sparsification of the graph and to train the proposed network. Finally, K-means is used to represent the latent features.

In our AHSGC, five clustering components are integrated into an end-to-end network for HSI clustering, and each part has interactions with the others.

6.3.2 HSI Preprocessing and Initial Graph Construction

In this chapter, initially, the simple linear iterative cluster (SLIC) [35] approach is utilized to partition the whole HSI into numerous spatially-connected superpixels. Subsequently, the superpixel-level node feature $\boldsymbol{X}$ is computed as the mean of the spectral features of the pixels within that superpixel. The matrix $\boldsymbol{A} \in \mathbb{R}^{N \times N}$ is defined as

$$\boldsymbol{A}_{ij} = \begin{cases} \mathrm{e}^{-\rho X_i - X_j^2}, \text{ if } \boldsymbol{X}_i \in N_t(\boldsymbol{X}_j) \text{ or } \boldsymbol{X}_j \in N_t(\boldsymbol{X}_i) \\ 0, \text{ otherwise} \end{cases} \tag{6.7}$$

where $\boldsymbol{X}_i$ represents the ith superpixel-level node feature, with $\rho = 0.2$, $N_t(\boldsymbol{X}_i)$ indicates the t-hop neighbors of the node v_i.

To investigate the relationship between pixel and superpixel, image backprojection operations are devised to convert data features from the pixel level to the superpixel level. This can be expressed as

$$\boldsymbol{Q}_{i,j} = \begin{cases} 1, \text{ if } x_i \in S_i \\ 0, \text{ otherwise} \end{cases} \tag{6.8}$$

where $\boldsymbol{Q} \in \mathbb{R}^{hw \times N}$ serves as the correlation matrix that keeps track of all the pixels in the HSI and their corresponding superpixels.

Graph projection has the ability to transform the original pixel-level HSI into superpixel-level graph node features via matrix multiplication. This process can be written as

$$\boldsymbol{V} = \text{Projection}(\boldsymbol{X}; \boldsymbol{Q}) = \hat{\boldsymbol{Q}}^T \text{Flatten}(\boldsymbol{X}) \tag{6.9}$$

where $\hat{\boldsymbol{Q}}$ is the column-normalized version of $\boldsymbol{Q}$, that is, $\hat{\boldsymbol{Q}}_{i,j} = \boldsymbol{Q}_{i,j} / \sum_m \boldsymbol{Q}_{m,j}$. The operation Flatten$(\cdot)$ implies flattening the HSI along the spatial dimensions, and the relevant equation can be presented as

6.3.3 Adaptive Filter Graph Encoder

Generally, low-pass filters can extract low-frequency information from the graph, filtering out high-frequency information, and thus obtaining smoother graph node signal features. In contrast, high-pass filters perform the opposite function (as shown in Fig. 6.2). Significantly, graph node signals consist of both low-pass and high-pass signals, and both have substantial effects on downstream clustering tasks [36]. Effectively leveraging these two types of feature signals is crucial for enhancing clustering accuracy.

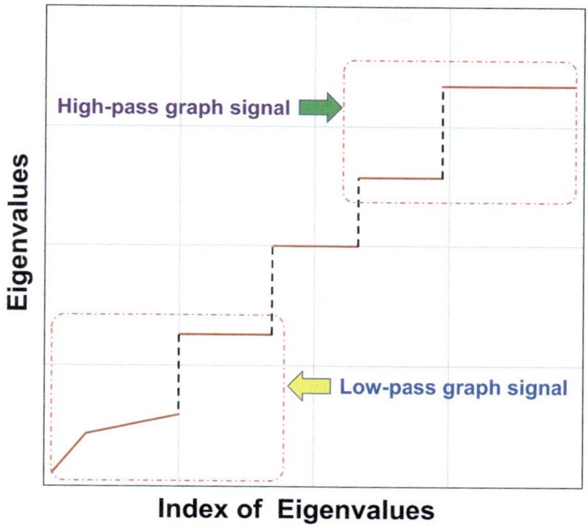

Fig. 6.2 Illustration of the role of low-pass and high-pass filters

In most cases, graph filters are respectively related to Laplacian matrices, affinity matrices, and their variations. The low-pass filters $\boldsymbol{H}_l$ and high-pass filters $\boldsymbol{H}_h$ can be represented as

$$\boldsymbol{H}_l = \boldsymbol{A}_{\mathrm{rw}}\boldsymbol{X}, \boldsymbol{H}_h = \boldsymbol{L}_{\mathrm{rw}}\boldsymbol{X} \tag{6.10}$$

where $\boldsymbol{A}_{rw}$ stands for the randomly wandering normalized affine matrix, which is formulated as $\boldsymbol{A}_{rw} = \boldsymbol{D}^{-1}\boldsymbol{A}$, $\boldsymbol{L}_{rw}$ is the corresponding Laplacian matrix, that is $\boldsymbol{L}_{rw} = \boldsymbol{I} - \boldsymbol{A}_{rw}$.

Based on the introduction in Sect. 6.2.1, when a convolution kernel f and a graph signal x are given, the convolution operation can be written as follows

$$f * x = \boldsymbol{U}\left(\left(\boldsymbol{U}^T f\right) \odot \left(\boldsymbol{U}^T x\right)\right) = \boldsymbol{U} g^\theta \boldsymbol{U}^T x \tag{6.11}$$

where $g^\theta = \boldsymbol{U}^T f$ indicates the representation of f in the spectral domain, and $\odot$ represents the matrix dot-product operation.

If $\boldsymbol{A}_{rw}$ and $\boldsymbol{L}_{rw}$ are regarded as convolution kernels according to Eq. (6.11), then we can filter the graph signal x as

$$\boldsymbol{A}_{rw} * x = \boldsymbol{U}\left(g_l^\theta\right)\boldsymbol{U}^T x, \boldsymbol{L}_{rw} * x = \boldsymbol{U}\left(g_h^\theta\right)\boldsymbol{U}^T x \tag{6.12}$$

where g_l^θ and g_h^θ stand for the spectral-domain representations of $\boldsymbol{A}_{rw}$ and $\boldsymbol{L}_{rw}$ respectively. Given that $g_l^\theta = \boldsymbol{I} - \boldsymbol{\Lambda}$ and $g_h^\theta = \boldsymbol{\Lambda}$, the Eq. (6.12) is rewrite as

$$\begin{aligned} U\left(g_l^{\theta}\right)\boldsymbol{U}^T x &= \sum_i (1-\lambda_i) u_i u_i^T x \\ U\left(g_h^{\theta}\right)\boldsymbol{U}^T x &= \sum_i \lambda_i u_i u_i^T x \end{aligned} \tag{6.13}$$

In Eq. (6.13), when the eigenvalue $\lambda > 1$, the disparities among the elements x_i are amplified in the projection $\sum_i \lambda_i u_i u_i^T x$, which enables the extraction of non-smooth signals. On the contrary, if $\lambda < 1$, the differences among x_i are diminished in the projection $\sum_i \lambda_i u_i u_i^T x$, allowing for the collection of smooth signals. Our analysis shows that low-pass filters are good at capturing similarity information, whereas high-pass filters perform the opposite task. Therefore, both types of filters are essential in graph networks. To comprehensively capture node information, we introduce an adaptive graph filter $\boldsymbol{F}_{\mathrm{A}}$, which is defined as

$$\boldsymbol{F}_{\mathrm{A}} = \mu \cdot (\boldsymbol{S}_{rw})^k \boldsymbol{X} + (1-\mu) \cdot (\boldsymbol{I} - \boldsymbol{S}_{rw})^k \boldsymbol{X} \tag{6.14}$$

where $\boldsymbol{X}$ represents the input spectral features, and $\mu > 0$ is a learnable parameter used to balance the high-pass and low-pass information. $\boldsymbol{S}_{rw}$ refers to the normalized Laplacian matrices related to $\boldsymbol{A}_{rw}$.

To acquire both high-pass and low-pass representations of the constructed graph, we stack t layers of graph Laplacian filters as shown below.

$$\boldsymbol{X}_s = \left(\prod_{i=1}^{t} \boldsymbol{F}_A\right)\boldsymbol{X} = \boldsymbol{F}_A^t \boldsymbol{X} \tag{6.15}$$

where $\boldsymbol{X}$ stands for the spectral features of the input graph nodes. $\boldsymbol{F}_A^t$ represents the stacked t layers of adaptive graph filters, and $\boldsymbol{X}_s$ indicates the representations of the graph nodes after t layers convolution.

6.3.4 *Graph Embedding Clustering Self-training Decoder*

(1) *Graph Embedding:* The adaptive filter graph encoder module is responsible for extracting high-level structural-semantic information, during which the high-pass and low-pass presentations are learned. In order to realize an effective fusion representation of structural information and spectral features, a linear transformation mechanism is designed to encode the graph structure as follows

$$\boldsymbol{Z} = \left(\prod_{i=1}^{t} \boldsymbol{F}_A\right)\boldsymbol{Z}_0 \boldsymbol{W} = \boldsymbol{F}_A^t \boldsymbol{Z}_0 \boldsymbol{W} \tag{6.16}$$

where $\boldsymbol{Z}_i$ and $\boldsymbol{Z}$ are the i-th layer and graph encoder output, respectively, $\boldsymbol{Z}_0 = \boldsymbol{X}$. The matrix $\boldsymbol{W}$ stands for the weight matrix of the linear transformation.

(2) *Self-Training Clustering:* As previously analyzed, we are able to learn high-pass and low-pass graph representations through an adaptive filter. Nevertheless, the high-level structural-semantic information cannot be directly applied to clustering, and the lack of labels poses an obstacle to graph clustering. To solve these issues, a self-training clustering mechanism is devised by making use of an auxiliary distribution. Specifically, we utilize a Student's t-distribution to gauge the similarity between the k-th cluster center $\boldsymbol{\mu}_k$ and the node embedding z_i as follows

$$q_{ik} = \frac{\left(1 + z_i - \mu_k^2\right)^{-1}}{\sum_k^K \left(1 + z_i - \mu_k^2\right)^{-1}} \tag{6.17}$$

where q_{ik} represents the clustering assignment distribution. It can be regarded as the soft assignment of node v_i to $\boldsymbol{\mu}_k$. Subsequently, we are able to optimize the clustering distribution by minimizing the KL divergence, that is

$$\mathcal{L}_c = KL(P\|Q) = \sum_i \sum_k p_{ik} \log \frac{p_{ik}}{q_{ik}} \tag{6.18}$$

$$p_{ik} = \frac{q_{ik}^2 / \sum_j q_{jk}}{\sum_k^K \left(q_{ik}^2 / \sum_j q_{jk}\right)} \tag{6.19}$$

where p_{ik} is the auxiliary distribution as detailed in Eq. (6.16), The operation of $\boldsymbol{P}$ on $\boldsymbol{Q}$ involves squaring $\boldsymbol{Q}$. This causes $\boldsymbol{Q}$ to become a more sharply defined distribution, thereby preventing the clustering from converging to a single cluster, as noted in [37].

6.3.5 Homophily-Enhanced Structure Learning

(1) *Orient Correlation Estimation:* When an intermediate clustering outcome is given, typically, the inner product is employed to measure the pairwise correlation between nodes. However, in actual practice, we've discovered that this method is not optimal. The reason is that the clustering results have a significant amount of noise during network training [38]. To tackle this issue, a hierarchical correlation estimation mechanism is devised. Specifically, the node similarity is estimated by integrating guidance from both the latent space in a hierarchical way and clustering. Initially, the hard pseudo-label is computed.

$$c_i = \arg\max_k q_{ik} \tag{6.20}$$

Based on Eq. (6.20), the pseudo-labels of all nodes are acquired. Subsequently, within each cluster k, the nodes' top γ with the highest assignment probability are chosen. As a result, a node subset is derived, specifically

$$\Gamma^k = \left\{ v_i | c_i = k, \text{Rank}|_{\{v_i|\mathrm{c_i=k}\}}(q_{ik}) \leq \gamma * |\{v_i|\mathrm{c_i = k}\}| \right\} \tag{6.21}$$

where Γ^k represents the top-confident node subset, and $\text{Rank}_{\{v_i|\mathrm{c_i=k}\}}(q_{ik})$ indicates the cluster assignment ranking probability of node v_i in cluster k. With Eq. (6.21), we can mitigate the impacts of noise on node clustering. Nevertheless, if the edge weight is still determined by the cluster space, segments that are confident but incorrect will still reduce the accuracy of the similarity matrix. To overcome these limitations, in this chapter, we use the latent space instead of the clustering space to estimate the node similarity.

In Eq. (6.16), the node embedding matrix $\boldsymbol{Z}$ is computed. We can then estimate the similarity between all nodes through the dot-product operation.

$$\boldsymbol{S} = \boldsymbol{Z}\boldsymbol{Z}^T \tag{6.22}$$

where $\boldsymbol{S}$ stands for the node similarity. Unlike in Eq. (6.22), in this chapter, we compute $\boldsymbol{S}$ within Γ^k. The corresponding node embedding node similarity $\boldsymbol{S}_{ij}^k$ is expressed as

$$\boldsymbol{S}_{ij}^k = \boldsymbol{Z}_i^k \boldsymbol{Z}_j^{k^T} \in \mathbb{R}^{|\Gamma^k| \times |\Gamma^k|} \tag{6.23}$$

where $\boldsymbol{Z}_i^k$ is the node embedding matrix of the i-th class, $\left|\Gamma^k\right|$ represents the quantity of nodes in Γ^k.

Equation (6.23) makes comprehensive use of the embedding similarity matrix and soft assignments to spot incorrect or missing edges. As a result, the accuracy of edge modification is notably improved. Thus, a more reliable and accurate graph structure learning can be realized.

(2) *Graph Edge Sparsification:* The majority of current methods maintain the graph in a static state during network training, that is, the edges within the graph do not change. This approach has two flaws. For example, incorrect edge connections in the graph cannot be rectified, and it poses unnecessary challenges for clustering. Taking inspiration from Eq. (6.6), we put forward a graph edge sparsification method. This method involves removing inter-cluster edges and recovering intra-cluster edges. The aim is to make the connections among nodes within a cluster closer and the connections between different clusters sparser (as illustrated in Fig. 6.3).

Intra-cluster edge recovery: In order to boost the connections within a cluster, edges are added to the top ξ percent of node pairs with the greatest similarity $\boldsymbol{S}_{ij}^k$ within cluster k, namely

$$\mathcal{E}_{rc}^k = \left\{ (v_i, v_j) \middle| \text{Rank}\left(\mathrm{S}_{ij}^k\right) \leq \xi * \left|\mathcal{E}\right| * \frac{N_k}{N}, \text{ and } c_i = c_j = k \right\} \tag{6.24}$$

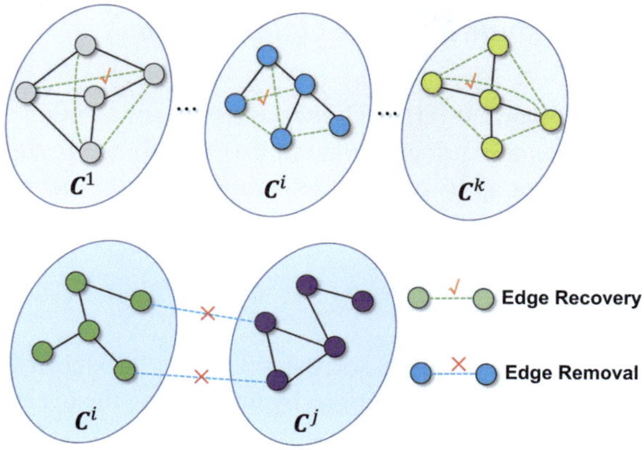

Fig. 6.3 The mechanism of intra-cluster edge recovery and Inter-cluster edge removal

$$\varepsilon_{rc} = \underset{k}{\overset{K}{U}} \varepsilon_{rc}^{k} \tag{6.25}$$

Inter-cluster edge removal: The objective of this approach is to get rid of needless edge links between clusters, reduce the connections among different clusters, and make clustering easier. The formula is presented as follows

$$\mathcal{E}_{rm} = \left\{ \left(v_i, v_j\right) \middle| \text{Rank}\left(\text{S}_{ij}\right) \geq (1-\eta)*|\mathcal{E}\;|, \left(v_i, v_j\right) \in \mathcal{E}, c_i \neq c_j \right\} \tag{6.26}$$

where $\mathcal{E}$ represents the edge-set in the current graph learning process. η is the proportion of edges to be retained.

(3) *Homophily-enhanced Structure Learning:* We have shown the edge sets for recovery and removal in Eqs. (6.25) and (6.26). The edge set during graph learning can be written as $\overline{\varepsilon} = \varepsilon - \varepsilon_{rm} + \varepsilon_{rc}$. The adjacency matrix $\overline{\boldsymbol{A}}$ can be computed as

$$\overline{\boldsymbol{A}} = \boldsymbol{A} - \boldsymbol{A}_{\mathcal{E}_{rm}} + \boldsymbol{A}_{\mathcal{E}_{rc}} \tag{6.27}$$

where $\boldsymbol{A}_{\mathcal{E}_{rm}}$ and $\boldsymbol{A}_{\mathcal{E}_{rc}}$ are the adjacency matrices corresponding to $\mathcal{E}_{rm}$ and $\mathcal{E}_{rc}$ respectively. Subsequently, we reconstruct the graph by renewing the adjacency matrix, specifically

$$\mathcal{L}_g = \boldsymbol{Z}\boldsymbol{Z}^T - \overline{\boldsymbol{A}}_F^2 \tag{6.28}$$

where $\mathcal{L}_g$ stands for the loss related to graph reconstruction.

This hierarchical approach overcomes the drawbacks of static graphs. It does so by dynamically adjusting the graph structure. As a result, nodes within the same cluster are more closely linked, and the unnecessary connections between different clusters are decreased.

6.3.6 Joint Network Optimization

In the proposed AHSGC, the losses of self-training clustering and structure graph reconstruction are presented in Eqs. (6.18) and (6.28), respectively. We utilize two loss functions to conduct self-training on the network and reconstruct the graph independently. Then, the overall objective $\mathcal{L}_O$ of AHSGC can be defined as

$$\mathcal{L}_O = \mathcal{L}_c + \mathcal{L}_g \tag{6.29}$$

In AHSGC, the p_{ik} is regarded as the "ground-truth". The hyper-parameters are updated through T iterations by minimizing the overall objective $\mathcal{L}_O$. The clustering outcome for node v_i is formulated as

$$Y_i = \underset{k}{\operatorname{argmax}}\, q_{ik} \tag{6.30}$$

Consequently, the adaptive filter graph encoder is employed to capture the latent features of the graph, from which the graph embeddings $\mathbf{Z}$ are obtained. After that, K-means is applied to conduct clustering on $\mathbf{Z}$ according to the initialized cluster centers $\boldsymbol{\mu}_k$. The learning procedure is elaborated in Algorithm 1.

Algorithm 1 AHSGC

```
Input: The input graph; Initial centroids (Cluster) number k; Iterations number T;
Number of the adaptive graph filter layer t.
Output: Clustering results Q.
Initialization: t; Z^0 = X;
Generate the homogeneous region and construct the superpixel-based graph;
for t = 1 to T do
        Apply t-layers graph convolution with adaptive graph filters on Z^0
        to obtain the latent Z by Eq. (6.16);
        The self-training clustering loss L_c is formulated as by Eq. (6.18);
        The homophily-enhanced structure learning is implemented by
        Eq. (6.24) and Eq. (6.26);
        The adjacency matrix Ā is calculated by Eq. (6.27);
        The graph reconstruction loss is calculated by Eq. (6.28)
        The weight matrices are updated by minimizing L_O with Adam
        optimizer.
end
The clustering results Q is obtained by applying K-means on Z.
```

6.4 Experimental Results

In this part, a series of comprehensive experiments and analyses are presented to evaluate the clustering performance of the proposed AHSGC. First, three well-known HSI datasets along with the experimental setups are described (in Sects. 6.4.1 and 6.4.2). Next, the quantitative and visual HSI clustering performances of AHSGC are contrasted with those of nine state-of-the-art algorithms (in Sects. 6.4.3 and 6.4.4). Then, the runtime and model complexity of AHSGC are compared with those of the investigated methods (in Sect. 6.4.5). Additionally, an analysis of the influence of hyperparameters is carried out (in Sect. 6.4.6). Moreover, clustering visualizations are shown (in Sect. 6.4.7). Finally, several ablation experiments are conducted to assess the rationality of the design of the proposed AHSGC (in Sect. 6.4.8).

6.4.1 Dataset Description

In this chapter, our method is validated by means of the Salina (SA), Trento, and Pavia University (PU) datasets. The SA dataset has dimensions of 512×217 and 204 bands, with a total of 16 land cover classes. The Trento dataset has an image size of 600×166 and 63 spectral channels spanning from 0.40 to 0.98 μm, covering 6 land cover classes. The PU dataset is an image with 103 spectral bands and dimensions of 610×340, including 9 land cover classes. Table 6.2 presents the specific land covers and their corresponding quantities for the three datasets, while the corresponding ground-truth is depicted in Fig. 6.4.

6.4.2 Experimental Setup

(1) *Experiment Settings:* The overall classification accuracy (OA), kappa coefficient (κ), normalized mutual information (NMI), adjusted rand index (ARI), and Purity are employed as quantitative assessment metrics. Specifically, OA serves to record the overall clustering precision; κ is an index utilized to assess the degree of consistency; NMI indicates the similarity of the clustering outcomes; ARI reflects the degree of agreement between the clustering results and the ground truth. Purity, which ranges from 0 to 1, is a straightforward and clear evaluation metric. In our AHSGC, seven key parameters need to be predefined. These are the number of graphs N, the number of encoder layers l, the number of iterations T, learning rate L, the intra-cluster edge recovery ratio ξ, the inter-cluster edge removal ratio η, and the high-confidence node extraction ratio γ. Their optimal values are presented in Table 6.3 and will be analyzed in Sect. 6.4.6.

Table 6.2 The details of each land-cover class of three datasets used in the chapter

No.	SA		PU		Trento	
	Name	Pixels	Name	Pixels	Name	Pixels
1	Weed 1	2009	Asphalt	6631	Apple trees	4034
2	Weed 2	3726	Meadows	18,649	Buildings	2903
3	Fallow	1976	Gravel	2099	Ground	479
4	Fallow-plow	1394	Trees	3064	Woods	9123
5	Fallow-smooth	2678	Painted metal sheets	1345	Vineyard	10,501
6	Stubble	3959	Bare Soil	5029	Roads	3174
7	Celery	3579	Bitumen	1330		
8	Grapes untrained	11,271	Self-Blocking Bricks	3682		
9	Soil	6203	Shadows	947		
10	Corn	3278				
11	Lettuce-4wk	1068				
12	Lettuce-5wk	1927				
13	Lettuce-6wk	916				
14	Lettuce-7wk	1070				
15	Vineyard-untrained	7268				
16	Vineyard-trellis	1807				
Total		54,129		42,776		30,214

(2) *Compare Baseline:* To thoroughly analyze the effectiveness of the proposed approach, we contrast AHSGC with nine chosen baselines, such as K-means, Fuzzy C-means (FCM), Possibilistic C-means (PCM), NCSC [18], DFCN [39], SDCN [40], EGAE [41], AdaGAE [42], and DAEGC [30]. Among these, K-means, FCM, and PCM are conventional clustering methods. NCSC and DAEGC are subspace clustering and graph clustering methods respectively. DFCN, SDCN, EGAE, AdaGAE, and DAEGC are deep clustering methods, while DAEGC, EGAE, and AdaGAE are graph autoencoder methods. The hyper-parameters and network structures of these methods adhere to the recommendations in the original papers.

(3) *Implementation details:* In this chapter, all the experiments under investigation are carried out on an NVIDIA Titan RTX using the Pytorch framework. For an equitable comparison, all methods are run ten times to eliminate any bias resulting from the random selection of training samples.

6.4.3 Quantitative and Qualitative Performances Comparison

In this part, we contrast AHSGC with nine other clustering techniques and demonstrate its clustering performance via both quantitative and qualitative performance

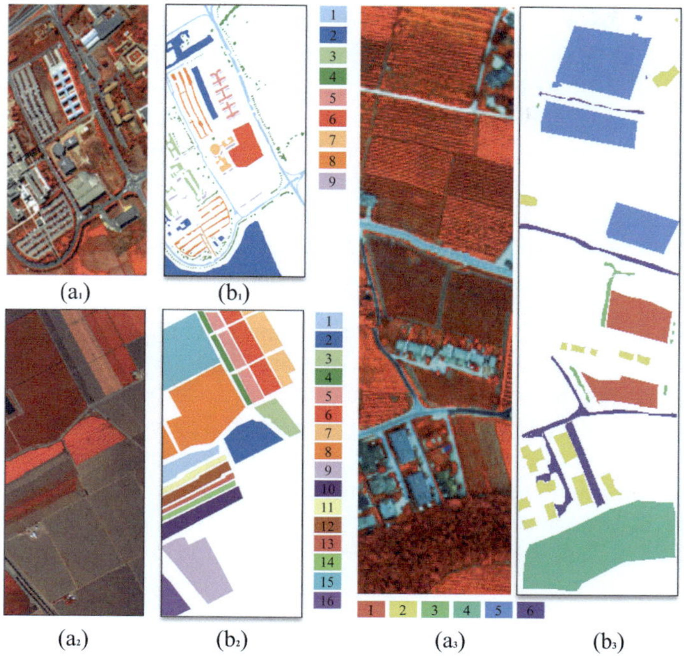

Fig. 6.4 Three dataset details. ($\mathbf{a_1}$), ($\mathbf{a_2}$), and ($\mathbf{a_3}$) are the false-color maps of SA, PU, and Trento datasets. ($\mathbf{b_1}$), ($\mathbf{b_2}$), and ($\mathbf{b_3}$) are the ground-truth maps

Table 6.3 Preset optimal parameters in AHSGC

Dataset	N	l	T	L	γ	ξ	η
Salinas	580	5	50	5e−4	0.3	0.5	0.05
PU	800	5	50	5e−4	0.5	0.5	0.05
Trento	550	5	50	5e−4	0.3	0.5	0.05

evaluations. Additionally, for greater intuitiveness, the top-performing results and the second-best results are indicated by bold and underlined formatting.

(1) *Quantitative analysis of the SA dataset:* The performances of various clustering methods on the SA dataset are presented in Table 6.4. As can be seen from Table 6.4, our AHSGC attains the optimal clustering performance, achieving 83.60%, 81.62%, 77.42%, and 83.68% in terms of OA, Kappa, NMI, ARI, and Purity respectively. This represents an improvement of 4.47%, 5.60%, 0.73%, 5.59%, and 0.11% when compared to the second-best outcomes. Moreover, NCSC, EGAE, and AdaGAE yield relatively favorable clustering results, indicating that these methods possess good adaptability to noise interference and the clustering of imbalanced class samples. Additionally, owing to the

significant capability of graph-based methods to utilize the inter-node relationships, DAEGC, EGAE, and AdaGAE manage to achieve relatively good clustering results. Because traditional methods such as k-mean, FCM, and PCM lack the ability to capture the high-level features of HSI, they inevitably produce poor results. Specifically, the OAs of these three methods are 67.99%, 56.73%, and 55.63% respectively. Furthermore, in comparison with other graph-based methods, an adaptive filter is capable of adaptively extracting both high-frequency and low-frequency information for subsequent HSI clustering tasks, thereby enhancing the performance of AHSGC.

(2) *Quantitative analysis of the PU dataset:* When contrasted with the SA dataset, the land cover types in the PU dataset are more spread out, presenting substantial difficulties for clustering. From the clustering outcomes shown in Table 6.5, it can also be deduced that the clustering results of all the compared methods have declined. Nevertheless, our AHSGC method still outperforms all the investigated clustering techniques. Significantly, in comparison to the best results among the comparative methods, the performances of AHSGC have increased by 3.55% in OA, 1.83% in κ, and 0.77% in ARI respectively. Moreover, we

Table 6.4 Quantitative experimental classification results on Salinas

No.	k-means	FCM	PCM	NCSC	DFCN	SDCN	EGAE	AdaGAE	DAEGC	AHSGC
1	0.9985	0.4179	0.6456	0.0000	**1.0000**	0.0000	**1.0000**	0.0000	**1.0000**	**1.0000**
2	0.5698	0.5524	0.8125	**1.0000**	0.9990	**1.0000**	**1.0000**	0.9997	0.9997	**1.0000**
3	0.9741	0.8501	0.0000	0.6822	**1.0000**	0.3426	**1.0000**	**1.0000**	0.0000	0.9413
4	**0.9865**	0.0000	0.0000	0.0000	0.0000	0.0000	0.0000	0.0000	0.0000	0.0000
5	0.7856	0.5540	0.9628	**0.9988**	0.7308	0.9816	0.0000	0.9572	0.6502	0.9709
6	0.9952	0.9990	0.9906	0.9941	0.9986	0.9530	0.9886	0.9900	**1.0000**	0.9914
7	0.4810	0.0000	0.9943	**1.0000**	0.9561	0.0000	0.9983	0.9999	0.9718	0.9922
8	0.7309	0.7772	0.3875	0.8026	0.4320	0.7633	0.5131	0.5631	0.6683	**0.9403**
9	0.9750	0.6969	0.5829	0.9076	0.9063	0.8643	0.8326	0.9832	0.9141	**0.9969**
10	0.6169	0.5507	0.4831	**0.9900**	0.7215	0.5519	0.8962	0.9000	0.2379	0.9356
11	0.3370	0.0000	0.7462	**0.9531**	0.5511	0.0000	0.0000	0.8702	0.0000	0.0000
12	0.0273	0.0047	0.8357	0.0000	0.5051	0.2287	**1.0000**	0.4926	0.8583	0.1012
13	0.3548	0.8134	**0.9582**	0.0000	0.0656	0.0690	0.0000	0.0000	0.0000	0.0000
14	0.5584	0.6512	0.1390	0.0000	0.0013	**0.7632**	0.0000	0.0000	0.0000	0.0000
15	0.4994	0.4279	0.2570	0.8563	0.9477	0.0980	**0.9692**	0.9436	0.8176	0.7881
16	0.0000	0.8321	0.4382	**1.0000**	0.2911	0.0000	**1.0000**	0.9575	0.9723	**1.0000**
OA (%)	0.6799	0.5673	0.5563	0.7881	0.7193	0.5382	0.7361	0.7683	0.7066	**0.8360**
Kappa	0.6572	0.5431	0.5472	0.7602	0.6900	0.4793	0.7106	0.7382	0.6741	**0.8162**
NMI	0.7356	0.6859	0.6631	0.8514	0.8288	0.6589	0.8769	0.8251	0.7841	**0.8587**
ARI	0.5466	0.4693	0.4539	0.7068	0.6278	0.4831	0.7183	0.6532	0.6096	**0.7742**
Purity	0.7132	0.7016	0.6708	0.7893	0.7324	0.5765	0.8357	0.8002	0.7129	**0.8368**

observe that deep and graph-based clustering methods do not have distinct advantages over traditional clustering methods. This is mainly because the land features in the PU dataset are dispersed and closely intertwined, making it hard for clustering methods to differentiate. As a result, extracting more prominent and representative features becomes more crucial. It is worthy of note that DAEGC and AHSGC have achieved remarkable performance, with OAs of 60.10% and 63.65% respectively. This is mainly because these two methods employ the structural graph learning mechanism, which can effectively learn the graph's structural information, meaning they have a better grasp of the graph's latent spatial structural details.

(3) *Quantitative analysis of the Trento dataset:* In comparison to the SA and PU datasets, the Trento dataset has a relatively uncomplicated distribution of land cover types. However, as seen in Table 6.6, the performance of traditional clustering methods such as k-means, FCM, and PCM is still disappointing. Their OAs are merely 63.01%, 51.32%, and 36.78% respectively, due to their limited feature extraction capabilities. Notably, AHSGC has obtained praiseworthy results, with an OA of 86.03%, surpassing the second-best performance by 10.41%. This is mainly attributable to its strong feature extraction ability and the discriminative power between different types of clusters. Thanks to the homophily-enhanced structure learning module, AHSGC can assess the relationships between nodes and classes, allowing for the automatic update of edge connections between nodes, thereby enhancing clustering accuracy. Additionally, the self-supervised structure and feature loss facilitate the self-representation feature extraction of HSI.

Table 6.5 Quantitative experimental classification results on PU

No.	*k*-means	FCM	PCM	NCSC	DFCN	SDCN	EGAE	AdaGAE	DAEGC	AHSGC
1	0.8234	0.5732	0.5538	0.4238	0.4051	0.6234	0.3029	**0.8521**	0.3759	0.4416
2	0.3581	0.3265	0.4633	0.5933	0.4008	0.3803	0.5012	0.5329	**0.7935**	0.7466
3	0.2167	0.0024	0.6027	0.6902	0.7038	0.1687	**0.9900**	0.7194	0.9609	0.4383
4	0.5943	0.5367	0.1648	0.0270	0.3547	0.4025	0.2744	**0.7237**	0.6505	0.6364
5	0.6620	0.7124	0.0000	0.9735	0.6892	0.6610	**1.0000**	0.0000	**1.0000**	**1.0000**
6	0.4255	0.3529	0.3265	0.9711	0.4940	0.3328	**1.0000**	0.4932	0.3327	0.4979
7	0.0000	**0.9578**	0.0068	0.3382	0.3486	0.3622	0.0000	0.0000	0.5301	0.6474
8	**0.9608**	0.8730	0.5538	0.4027	0.3444	0.4729	0.6258	0.2320	0.1645	0.7588
9	**0.9990**	0.0000	0.9989	0.0000	0.1683	0.3702	0.0000	0.4538	0.0847	0.0000
OA (%)	0.5237	0.4359	0.4376	0.5519	0.4214	0.4207	0.5328	0.5436	0.6010	**0.6365**
Kappa	0.5246	0.4327	0.4261	0.4570	0.3189	0.3185	0.4536	0.4139	0.4866	**0.5429**
NMI	**0.5529**	0.5126	0.4758	0.4392	0.4355	0.4362	0.5372	0.4628	0.5142	0.5251
ARI	0.3188	0.2632	0.2783	0.3869	0.2691	0.2399	0.3780	0.3271	0.5049	**0.5128**
Purity	**0.7012**	0.6785	0.6487	0.6638	0.5966	0.6400	0.7126	0.6689	0.6842	0.6980

Table 6.6 Quantitative experimental classification results on Trento

No.	*k*-means	FCM	PCM	NCSC	DFCN	SDCN	EGAE	AdaGAE	DAEGC	AHSGC
1	0.0000	0.0000	0.3673	**1.0000**	0.6844	0.2218	0.6522	**1.0000**	**1.0000**	0.9995
2	0.0189	0.0000	0.0000	0.0793	0.4191	0.7826	0.6029	0.4826	0.1151	**1.0000**
3	0.0000	0.0000	0.0000	0.0000	0.0063	0.0359	**0.0931**	0.0000	0.0000	0.0000
4	0.7200	0.6826	0.4502	**1.0000**	0.9745	0.6237	0.9540	0.9622	**1.0000**	**1.0000**
5	0.6182	0.2007	0.4292	0.6437	0.7105	0.7452	0.5196	0.6158	0.6156	**0.9394**
6	0.0199	0.0329	0.0006	0.8206	0.3959	0.5930	0.3412	0.8029	**0.8233**	0.0224
OA (%)	0.6301	0.5132	0.3678	0.7489	0.7145	0.6200	0.6487	0.7562	0.7469	**0.8603**
Kappa	0.6026	0.4917	0.3232	0.6790	0.6314	0.5132	0.5380	0.6810	0.6741	**0.8148**
NMI	0.4928	0.4654	0.2898	0.7312	0.6787	0.4860	0.6801	0.7250	0.6767	**0.8844**
ARI	0.3457	0.2802	0.1303	0.7111	0.6795	0.4362	0.6624	0.6455	0.6483	**0.8884**
Purity	0.6499	0.6708	0.5146	0.8652	0.7817	0.7050	0.8273	0.7726	0.8382	**0.8810**

6.4.4 Visual Clustering Results Analysis

To present the clustering results in a visual manner, various colormaps are utilized to signify the clustering outcomes of different land features, as depicted in Figs. 6.5, 6.6 and 6.7. From these visualized clustering results, it can be inferred that the clustering outcomes of traditional methods like *K*-means, FCM, and PCM are rife with salt-and-pepper noise. This indicates their inadequate feature extraction capabilities and poor noise resilience. Owing to their capacity for nonlinear representation and high-level feature extraction, deep-learning methods yield smoother colormaps with reduced noise. Nevertheless, for particular details such as edge pixels, misclassifications might take place. Thanks to the adaptive filter, AHSGC is able to effectively capture both low-pass and high-pass information for clustering purposes, and the excessive high-frequency and low-frequency noises are filtered out. Moreover, the homophily-enhanced structure learning module, through estimating the edge connections between nodes and classes, can update the connections among nodes and those between classes. As a result, the perceptual representation of the HSI topology is effectively captured.

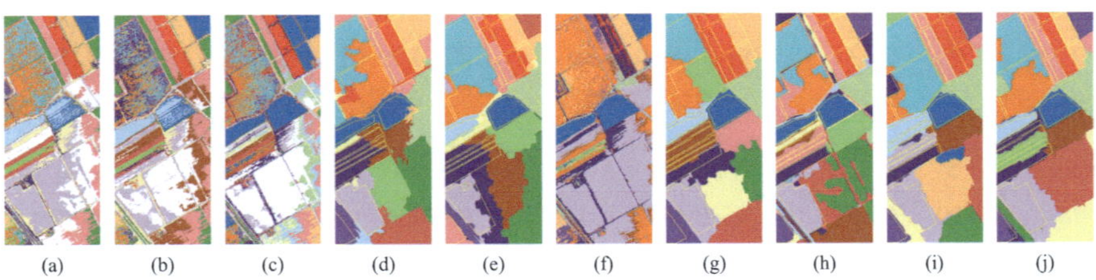

Fig. 6.5 Clustering maps of SA dataset. **a** K-means, **b** FCM, **c** PCM, **d** NCSC, **e** DFCN, **f** SDCN, **g** EGAE, **h** AdaGAE, **i** DAEGC, **j** AHSGC

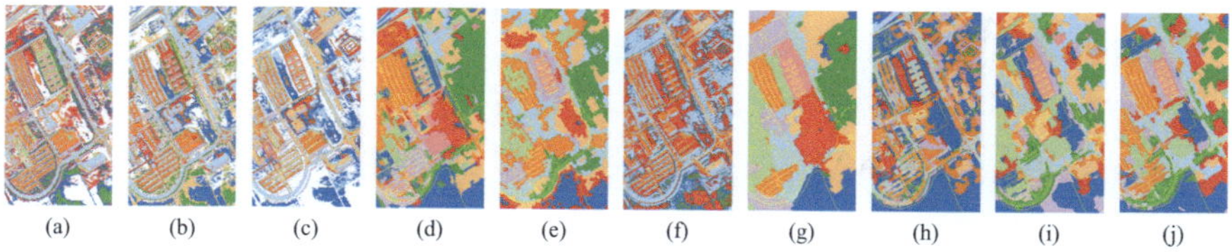

Fig. 6.6 Clustering maps of PU dataset. **a** K-means, **b** FCM, **c** PCM, **d** NCSC, **e** DFCN, **f** SDCN, **g** EGAE, **h** AdaGAE, **i** DAEGC, **j** AHSGC

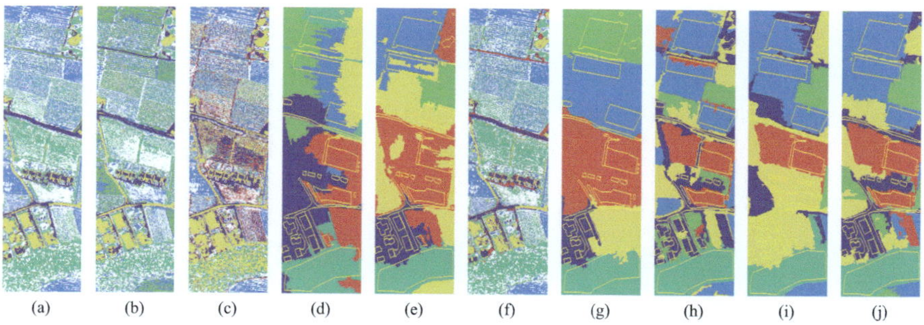

Fig. 6.7 Clustering maps of Trento dataset. **a** K-means, **b** FCM, **c** PCM, **d** NCSC, **e** DFCN, **f** SDCN, **g** EGAE, **h** AdaGAE, **i** DAEGC, **j** AHSGC

6.4.5 Complexity Comparison

In this section, we evaluate the runtime and model complexity of all the deep clustering methods under study. We document the indices of training time, testing time, and FLOP to contrast the computational cost and model complexity among different methods. As per the results presented in Table 6.7, we observe that the training time, testing time, and model complexity of our method are considerably lower than those of other investigated methods, validating the effectiveness of HSI processing. Additionally, because of the potent and rapid feature extraction capabilities of AHSGC, which only needs 50 epochs to reach convergence, its training time is relatively brief. Moreover, AHSGC employs task-oriented self-training and graph structure reconstruction objective loss to effectively enhance the acceleration ability. As a result, the representative features are extracted and the computational efficiency of the model is improved. Thus, we can infer that our method attains outstanding clustering results with a relatively low model complexity, suggesting that AHSGC holds excellent practical application prospects.

Table 6.7 The running time and model complexity of all deep clustering methods on three datasets

Name	Salinas			PU			Trento		
	Train/s	Test/s	FLOPs	Train/s	Test/s	FLOPs	Train/s	Test/s	FLOPs
AdaGAE	144.8671	43.5324	130.02 M	1200.819	101.3368	1.29G	86.2017	13.7605	25.53 M
EAGE	199.946	4.8399	270.38 M	1763.686	39.8889	2.63G	186.1897	4.7581	57.09 M
NCSC	681.0274	15.6768	303.18G	1375.568	33.2784	596.49G	677.5501	19.3583	273.67G
DAEGC	73.4302	5.1500	148.72 M	581.7761	44.8480	1.46 G	65.9399	4.7916	27.75 M
DFCN	672.1873	4.2803	490.69 M	1802.5410	8.5483	1.70 G	282.6037	4.4386	83.27 M
SDCN	437.5881	0.6087	446.1G	274.8834	0.2034	339.56G	145.6749	0.3492	236.22G
AHSGC	179.9025	0.0025	3.57 G	237.5779	0.0007	30.62G	56.2532	0.0629	2.95 G

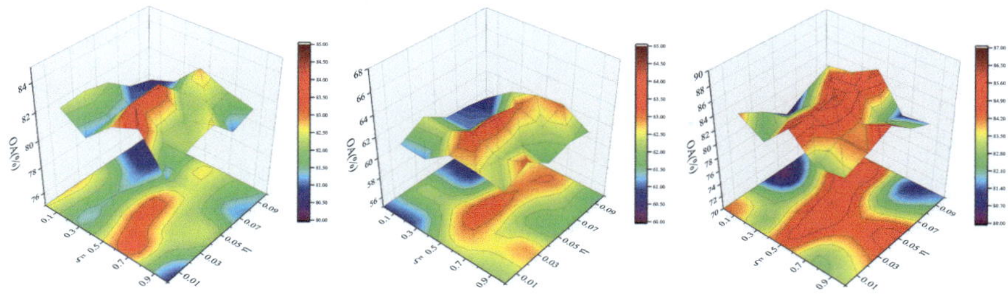

Fig. 6.8 Sensitivities of ξ and η on SA (**a**), PU (**b**), and Trento (**c**)

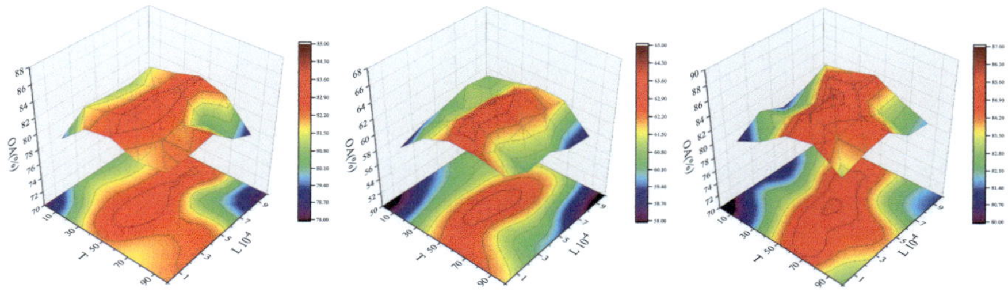

(a) (b) (c)

Fig. 6.9 Sensitivities of T and L on SA (**a**), PU (**b**), and Trento (**c**)

6.4.6 Parameter Analysis

In this part, an investigation is carried out on the effects of diverse hyperparameters within AHSGC on the clustering performance. The number of iterations T, learning rate L, intra-cluster edge recovery ratio ξ, and inter-cluster edge removal ratio η are explored through a grid search strategy. Fig. 6.8 and Fig. 6.9 illustrate the changes in OA across three datasets corresponding to different values of (ξ, η) and (T, L), respectively. From these results, it can be seen that the four parameters have a substantial influence on the final clustering accuracy. Moreover, the model has a higher likelihood of attaining superior performance when $\in [0.5, 0.7]$, $\eta \in [0.3, 0.5]$, $T \in [40, 60]$, and $L \in \left[3\mathrm{e}^{-4}, 5\mathrm{e}^{-4}\right]$, respectively.

6.4.7 Clustering Visualization

In this segment, the *t*-distributed stochastic neighbor embedding (t-SNE) [43] technique is utilized to visualize the distribution of graph nodes in three datasets for validating the clustering performance of AHSGC. In Fig. 6.10a–c display the original distribution of the initial graph nodes, whereas (d)–(f) depict the distribution of graph

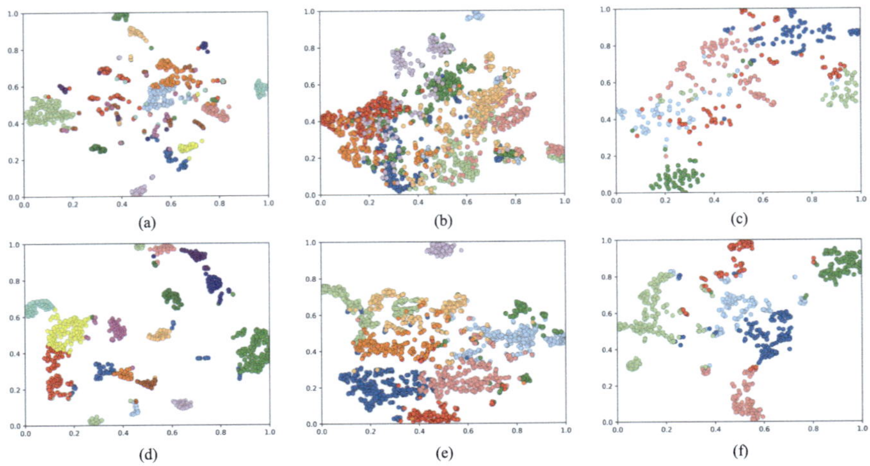

Fig. 6.10 Visualizing AHSGC with t-SNE on the SA dataset in **a** and **d**, the PU dataset in **b** and **e**, and the Trento dataset in **c** and **f**. The distributions in **a**, **b**, and **c** pertain to the original states of the three datasets. Those in **d**, **e**, and **f** represent the distributions following the clustering process. Nodes of distinct colors within these maps stand for different land cover types

node features subsequent to processing with AHSGC. Through comparison and analysis, the following inferences can be made: (1) The distribution covariance among different classes in (d)–(f) is lower than that in (a)–(c), signifying that favorable clustering outcomes have been achieved; (2) Compared to (a)–(c), (d)–(f) exhibit greater inter-class distances and smaller intra-class distances, presenting a more ordered and compact distribution; (3) Different land cover types are more distinctly differentiated. Consequently, graph nodes processed by AHSGC show stronger intra-class compactness and larger inter-class distances. Moreover, the clustering task described in Eq. (6) is effectively carried out.

6.4.8 Ablation Experiment

In this part, we are going to assess the role of the adaptive filter graph encoder, homophily-enhanced structure learning, as well as the HSI preprocessing and initial graph construction module in the overall clustering performance. Moreover, a series of ablation experiments have been carried out. Specifically, AHSGC without the homogeneous regions generation block is named AHSGC-V1. AHSGC-V2 is created by eliminating the adaptive filter graph encoder block. AHSGC-V3 is derived by removing the homophily-enhanced structure learning block. The outcomes are presented in Fig. 6.11, which records five metrics. From these results, we can observe that different modules in AHSGC have varying effects on clustering accuracy. Also, every module in AHSGC plays a part in enhancing the clustering accuracy.

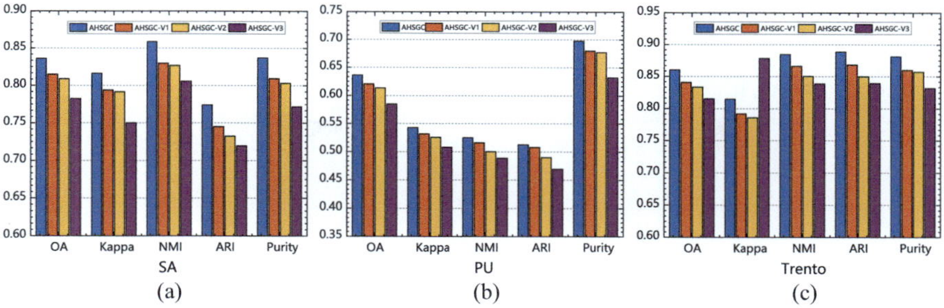

Fig. 6.11 Ablation experiment results with five metrics on three datasets

6.5 Conclusion

In this chapter, a new homophily-enhanced structure graph learning approach combined with an adaptive filter clustering method (AHSGC) for HSI is put forward. In detail, a homogeneous region generation technique is utilized to preprocess the HSI. This helps in preserving the local spatial-spectral structure information and simultaneously reduces the number of nodes in the graph. Subsequently, an adaptive filter graph encoder is incorporated to adaptively capture both high- and low-frequency features on the graph for the clustering task. Next, a graph embedding clustering self-training decoder is developed using KL Divergence, which generates pseudo-labels for network training. At the same time, a homophily-enhanced structure graph learning module is designed to update the graph based on the task. In this module, the orient correlation estimation is employed to estimate node connections, and graph edge sparsification is designed to dynamically adjust the edges within the graph. Finally, joint network optimization is proposed to optimize the network, and K-means is used to represent the latent features.

Regarding future work, several additional spatial-spectral self-supervised methods will be investigated for graph learning. Moreover, some further research, such as reinforcement learning, will be applied to HSI preprocessing to improve the feature extraction capabilities of clustering methods.

References

1. Peng J, Sun W, Du Q (2018) Self-paced joint sparse representation for the classification of hyperspectral images. IEEE Trans Geosci Remote Sens 57(2):1183–1194
2. Peng J, Li L, Tang YY (2018) Maximum likelihood estimation-based joint sparse representation for the classification of hyperspectral remote sensing images. IEEE Trans Neural Netw Learn Syst 30(6):1790–1802
3. Lv Z, Huang H, Sun W, Lei T, Benediktsson JA, Li J (2023) Novel enhanced UNet for change detection using multimodal remote sensing image. IEEE Geosci Remote Sens Lett 20:1–5

4. Lv Z, Liu J, Sun W, Lei T, Benediktsson JA, Jia X (2023) Hierarchical attention feature fusion-based network for land cover change detection with homogeneous and heterogeneous remote sensing images. IEEE Trans Geosci Remote Sens 61:1–15
5. Feng J, Bai G, Li D, Zhang X, Shang R, Jiao L (2022) MR-selection: A meta-reinforcement learning approach for zero-shot hyperspectral band selection. IEEE Trans Geosci Remote Sens 61:1–20
6. Feng J, Chen J, Sun Q, Shang R, Cao X, Zhang X, Jiao L (2020) Convolutional neural network based on bandwise-independent convolution and hard thresholding for hyperspectral band selection. IEEE Trans Cybern 51(9):4414–4428
7. Yao D, Zhi-li Z, Xiao-feng Z, Wei C, Fang H, Yao-ming C, Cai W-W (2023) Deep hybrid: multi-graph neural network collaboration for hyperspectral image classification. Defence Technol 23:164–176
8. Lou C, Al-qaness MA, AL-Alimi D, Dahou A, Abd Elaziz M, Abualigah L, Ewees AA (2024) Land use/land cover (LULC) classification using hyperspectral images: a review. Geo-spatial Inform Sci 1–42
9. Cai Y, Zhang Z, Liu X, Ding Y, Li F, Tan J (2024) Learning unified anchor graph for joint clustering of hyperspectral and LiDAR data. IEEE Trans Neural Netw Learn Syst 36(4):6341–6354
10. Ding Y, Zhao X, Zhang Z, Cai W, Yang N (2021) Graph sample and aggregate-attention network for hyperspectral image classification. IEEE Geosci Remote Sens Lett 19:1–5
11. Ding Y, Zhang Z, Zhao X, Cai W, Yang N, Hu H, Huang X, Cao Y, Cai W (2022) Unsupervised self-correlated learning smoothy enhanced locality preserving graph convolution embedding clustering for hyperspectral images. IEEE Trans Geosci Remote Sens 60:1–16
12. Dalal A-A, Al-qaness MA, Cai Z, Alawamy EA (2023) IDA: Improving distribution analysis for reducing data complexity and dimensionality in hyperspectral images. Pattern Recogn 134:109096
13. Kanungo T, Mount DM, Netanyahu NS, Piatko CD, Silverman R, Wu AY (2002) An efficient k-means clustering algorithm: analysis and implementation. IEEE Trans Pattern Anal Mach Intell 24(7):881–892
14. Yang X, Zhu M, Sun B, Wang Z, Nie F (2023) Fuzzy c-multiple-means clustering for hyperspectral image. IEEE Geosci Rem Sens Lett 20:1–5
15. Ng A, Jordan M, Weiss Y (2001) On spectral clustering: analysis and an algorithm. In Advances in neural information processing systems, vol 14
16. Krishnapuram R, Keller JM (1996) The possibilistic c-means algorithm: insights and recommendations. IEEE Trans Fuzzy Syst 4(3):385–393
17. Rodriguez A, Laio A (2014) Clustering by fast search and find of density peaks. Science 344(6191):1492–1496
18. Cai Y, Zhang Z, Ghamisi P, Ding Y, Liu X, Cai Z, Gloaguen R (2022) Superpixel contracted neighborhood contrastive subspace clustering network for hyperspectral images. IEEE Trans Geosci Remote Sens 60:1–13
19. Peng X, Tang H, Zhang L, Yi Z, Xiao S (2015) A unified framework for representation-based subspace clustering of out-of-sample and large-scale data. IEEE Trans Neural Netw Learn Syst 27(12):2499–2512
20. Gillis N, Kuang D, Park H (2014) Hierarchical clustering of hyperspectral images using rank-two nonnegative matrix factorization. IEEE Trans Geosci Remote Sens 53(4):2066–2078
21. Peng J, Sun W, Li H-C, Li W, Meng X, Ge C, Du Q (2021) Low-rank and sparse representation for hyperspectral image processing: a review. IEEE Geosci Remote Sens Mag 10(1):10–43
22. Su Y, Gao L, Jiang M, Plaza A, Sun X, Zhang B (2022) NSCKL: Normalized spectral clustering with kernel-based learning for semisupervised hyperspectral image classification. IEEE Trans Cybern 53(10):6649–6662
23. Zhang H, Bruzzone L, Shi W, Hao M, Wang Y (2018) Enhanced spatially constrained remotely sensed imagery classification using a fuzzy local double neighborhood information c-means clustering algorithm. IEEE J Select Top Appl Earth Observ Remote Sens 11(8):2896–2910

24. Zhai H, Zhang H, Zhang L, Li P, Plaza A (2016) A new sparse subspace clustering algorithm for hyperspectral remote sensing imagery. IEEE Geosci Remote Sens Lett 14(1):43–47
25. Wang R, Nie F, Wang Z, He F, Li X (2019) Scalable graph-based clustering with nonnegative relaxation for large hyperspectral image. IEEE Trans Geosci Remote Sens 57(10):7352–7364
26. Ding Y, Zhang Z, Zhao X, Hong D, Cai W, Yu C, Yang N, Cai W (2022) Multi-feature fusion: Graph neural network and CNN combining for hyperspectral image classification. Neurocomputing 501:246–257
27. Zhang Y, Wang Y, Chen X, Jiang X, Zhou Y (2022) Spectral–spatial feature extraction with dual graph autoencoder for hyperspectral image clustering. IEEE Trans Circuits Syst Video Technol 32(12):8500–8511
28. Ding Y, Zhang Z, Zhao X, Cai Y, Li S, Deng B, Cai W (2022) Self-supervised locality preserving low-pass graph convolutional embedding for large-scale hyperspectral image clustering. IEEE Trans Geosci Remote Sens 60:1–16
29. Luo F, Liu Y, Duan Y, Guo T, Zhang L, Du B (2024) SDST: self-supervised double-structure transformer for hyperspectral images clustering. IEEE Trans Geosci Remote Sens 62:1–14
30. Wang C, Pan S, Hu R, Long G, Jiang J, Zhang C (2019) Attributed graph clustering: a deep attentional embedding approach. arXiv preprint arXiv:1906.06532
31. Peng S, Yin J, Yang Z, Chen B, Lin Z (2023) Multiview clustering via hypergraph induced semi-supervised symmetric nonnegative matrix factorization. IEEE Trans Circuits Syst Video Technol 33(10):5510–5524
32. Chen Z, Wu G, Gao H, Ding Y, Hong D, Zhang B (2023) Local aggregation and global attention network for hyperspectral image classification with spectral-induced aligned superpixel segmentation. Expert Syst Appl 232:120828
33. Gu M, Yang G, Zhou S, Ma N, Chen J, Tan Q, Liu M, Bu J. Homophily-enhanced structure learning for graph clustering, pp 577–586
34. Wen Z, Ling Y, Ren Y, Wu T, Chen J, Pu X, Hao Z, He L (2024) Homophily-related: adaptive hybrid graph filter for multi-view graph clustering, pp 15841–15849
35. Achanta R, Shaji A, Smith K, Lucchi A, Fua P, Süsstrunk S (2012) SLIC superpixels compared to state-of-the-art superpixel methods. IEEE Trans Pattern Anal Mach Intell 34(11):2274–2282
36. Yang W, Mirzasoleiman B (2023) Contrastive learning under heterophily. arXiv preprint arXiv: 2303.06344
37. Pan E, Kang Z (2023) Beyond homophily: reconstructing structure for graph-agnostic clustering. In: International conference on machine learning. PMLR, pp 26868–26877
38. Liu Y, Yang X, Zhou S, Liu X, Wang S, Liang K, Tu W, Li L (2023) Simple contrastive graph clustering. IEEE Trans Neural Netw Learn Syst 35:13789–13800
39. Tu W, Zhou S, Liu X, Guo X, Cai Z, Zhu E, Cheng J (2021) Deep fusion clustering network. AAAI Conf Artif Intell 35(11):9978–9987
40. Bo D, Wang X, Shi C, Zhu M, Lu E, Cui P (2020) Structural deep clustering network. In: Proceedings of the web conference, pp 1400–1410
41. Zhang H, Li P, Zhang R, Li X (2022) Embedding graph auto-encoder for graph clustering. IEEE Trans Neural Netw Learn Syst 34(11):9352–9362
42. Li X, Zhang H, Zhang R (2021) Adaptive graph auto-encoder for general data clustering. IEEE Trans Pattern Anal Mach Intell 44(12):9725–9732
43. Van der Maaten L, Hinton G (2008) Visualizing data using t-SNE. J Mach Learn Res 9(11)

MIX
Papier aus verantwortungsvollen Quellen
Paper from responsible sources
FSC® C105338

If you have any concerns about our products,
you can contact us on
ProductSafety@springernature.com

In case Publisher is established outside the EU,
the EU authorized representative is:
Springer Nature Customer Service Center GmbH
Europaplatz 3, 69115 Heidelberg, Germany

Printed by Libri Plureos GmbH
in Hamburg, Germany